Redleaf
3/31/10
$37.95

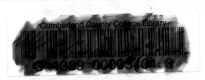
Cumberland County College Library
34399 00005404 8

W9-BZK-798

Rethinking Nutrition

JUL X X 2015

WITHDRAWN

Also in This Series:

*Intellectual Development:*
*Connecting Science and Practice in Early Childhood Settings*

*Social and Emotional Development:*
*Connecting Science and Practice in Early Childhood Settings*

CUMBERLAND COUNTY COLLEGE LIBRARY
PO BOX 1500
VINELAND, NJ 08362-1500

# Rethinking Nutrition

Connecting Science and Practice
in Early Childhood Settings

Susan Nitzke, PhD, RD

Dave Riley, PhD

Ann Ramminger, MS

Georgine Jacobs, MS

with Ellen Sullivan, RD, MS, CD

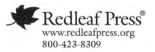

**Redleaf Press®**
www.redleafpress.org
800-423-8309

RJ
206
R48
2010

Published by Redleaf Press
10 Yorkton Court
St. Paul, MN 55117
www.redleafpress.org

© 2010 by Susan Nitzke, Dave Riley, Ann Ramminger, and Georgine Jacobs

All rights reserved. Unless otherwise noted on a specific page, no portion of this publication may be reproduced or transmitted in any form or by any means, electronic or mechanical, including photocopying, recording, or capturing on any information storage and retrieval system, without permission in writing from the publisher, except by a reviewer, who may quote brief passages in a critical article or review to be printed in a magazine or newspaper, or electronically transmitted on radio, television, or the Internet.

First edition 2010
Cover design by Jim Handrigan
Interior typeset in Sabon
Photo on page 89 courtesy of Andrew Nitzke
Photos on pages 36 and 90 courtesy of William Nitzke
Photos on pages 9, 11, and 17 courtesy of Georgine Jacobs
Photo on page 57 courtesy of Mary Ann Rinkleff
Printed in the United States of America

17  16  15  14  13  12  11  10      1 2 3 4 5 6 7 8

Library of Congress Cataloging-in-Publication Data

Rethinking nutrition : connecting science and practice in early childhood settings / Susan Nitzke ... [et al.].—1st ed.
    p. cm.
Includes bibliographical references and index.
ISBN 978-1-60554-031-3 (alk. paper)
1.  Children—Nutrition.  I. Nitzke, Susan A.
RJ206.R48 2010
618.92'39—dc22
                                    2009049715


Printed on acid-free paper

We dedicate this book to

farmers and gardeners, who produce good food,
upon which all else matters;

cooks, who make food into tastes that add art to our lives;

hosts, who stimulate gatherings and conversations,
creating community from the necessity for nourishment;

children, who inspire us with their curiosity,
excitement, and smiles; and

great early childhood programs,
which include all four of these.

# Rethinking Nutrition

# Preface

This book is part of a series that is unique because it was written by a team of academic researchers and early childhood program practitioners with common interests. In this case, the uniting interests are nutrition and its role as a key determinant of young children's overall well-being and prospects for lifelong health. We have chosen this book as our vehicle to share the science- and practice-based information we have assembled to help you—the early childhood teacher, administrator, or care provider—nurture young lives.

Each chapter begins with a summary of important concepts based on current scientific research and with recommendations from expert professional organizations. The research information is followed by a series of examples (practice tips, promising practices, and, in some cases, mistaken practices) that bring nutrition principles to life in early childhood settings. Near the end of each chapter are lists of further readings. We also include "When Teachers Reflect" sections, which have topic suggestions for staff discussions, and examples of letters to families that may be incorporated into newsletters, mailed letters, or online postings. The appendixes include practical resources that support and complement content in the book's five chapters. References cited in the text can be found after the appendixes.

Throughout *Rethinking Nutrition*, we randomly refer to individual children as "he" or "she" to avoid gender bias. We also use terms such as "caregiver," "teacher," and "early childhood professional" interchangeably to be inclusive of roles played by adults in early childhood settings.

# Acknowledgments

We wish to thank the following colleagues, who served as reviewers or provided helpful input during the preparation of this book. They truly helped us make this a better book.

- Ellyn Satter, MS, RD, LCSW, BCD, author, publisher, consultant, family therapist

- Madeleine Sigman-Grant, PhD, RD, University of Nevada Cooperative Extension

- Carol Philipps, MS, RD, Wisconsin Department of Public Instruction (retired)

- Mary Marcus, MS, RD, pediatric dietitian, UW Health American Family Children's Hospital

- Angela Nitzke Martin, MSJ, journalist

- Paula Ries, BS, director, University City United Church Preschool

- Amy Meinen, MPH, RD, Wisconsin Department of Health Services

- Barbara Ingham, PhD, professor and extension specialist, University of Wisconsin-Madison Food Science

We also express our appreciation to the editorial staff at Redleaf Press, who helped make this book a reality.

# 1

# Nutrition to Support Healthy Growth

## Observation: Tanya Wouldn't Eat Breakfast

*A father bustles into the child care room carrying his toddler-aged daughter in his arms and heads right over to the lead teacher, Maria. "We couldn't get Tanya to eat anything solid this morning," he reports. "We wrote down what she's eaten since last night," he says and hands teacher Maria a note. "No need to worry, Jim," Maria says, as she begins unzipping Tanya's jacket. "Toddlers can be finicky. It doesn't mean she's sick or anything. But we'll keep a close watch on what she eats and give you a call if she doesn't seem well."*

## Nutritional Needs

When parents leave their child at an early childhood program, their top concern is usually the child's safety and health. They want their child to be happy, make friends, and learn things, of course, but physical safety and health come first. Like the worried father in the introductory observation, parents have protective instincts that can make them worry. Good early childhood programs are comprehensive, meaning they deal with the whole child, including social-emotional development, intellectual development, and physical development.

Nutrition has strong and long-lasting effects on children's development. Good childhood nutrition helps children learn better and promotes strong, healthy bodies. In addition, eating habits and taste preferences formed in early childhood become the basis for lifelong eating behaviors. Just as with other aspects of child development, such as early language learning and emotional attachment, patterns established in the early years of life predict who will and who will not be healthy in the years ahead. The early childhood period is that crucial!

But aren't children's health and growth determined by their genetics? Certainly, much about a person's health is determined by biological inheritance, and much is also determined by early experiences. Other than the preference for sweet flavors, which is inborn in all humans, babies' taste preferences begin to take shape very early and are based on experiences months before they directly taste solid food. Even prior to birth, the mother's diet introduces flavors to the baby via the amniotic fluid that surrounds the fetus and gets swallowed while the baby is still in the womb. After birth, many flavors from the mother's diet are present in her breast milk. As children begin to eat at the family table and with other children in child care settings, they become familiar with an ever-widening variety of tastes and textures. Through this process, they form strong and lasting opinions about what foods and beverages are proper and preferred for meals, snacks, and celebrations.

## Birth to Six Months

By six months of age, most healthy babies weigh at least twice as much as they did at birth. Their brains, organs, bones, and other body tissues are developing at a rapid pace. Breast milk is the best source of nutrients during this period. The American Academy of Pediatrics (AAP) recommends breast-feeding as the only source of food for infants up to ages four to six months and encourages breast-feeding along with some semi-solid foods for the rest of the first year. The AAP states the following:

> Although economic, cultural and political pressures often confound decisions about infant feeding, the AAP firmly adheres to the position that breastfeeding ensures the best possible health as well as the best developmental and psychosocial outcomes for the infant.
>
> (American Academy of Pediatrics 2005, 501)

Breast milk contains antibodies that help build the baby's immunity to some common diseases, such as ear and intestinal infections. Breast milk contains the optimal balance of nutrients to promote brain and nervous system growth. Breast-feeding allows the infant to determine how much milk is consumed, based on the baby's internal feelings of hunger or satiety, which helps maintain the child's ability to self-regulate food intake and avoid overeating. Otherwise, overeating can become a habit that may lead to obesity in some children. In addition, the breast-feeding experience promotes close mother-child bonding, which is so important for the infant's social development.

## Be Breast-Feeding Friendly

Early childhood programs can do much to support, or interfere with, a mother's ability to continue breast-feeding. Some mothers choose to breast-feed at the child care facility, others provide their breast milk in bottles, and many find a combination that fits their needs. The following practices are recommended to promote breast-feeding and safely handle breast milk in early childhood programs:

- Provide a private room or nook with a comfortable chair, a pillow, and a step stool to make breast-feeding more comfortable for mother and baby. A place to wash hands should be nearby.

- Develop a feeding schedule that accommodates the mother's needs. She may want you to schedule the baby's feeding so that the baby is hungry and ready to breast-feed when she comes to get the baby.

- Have a refrigerator/freezer with adequate space devoted to breast milk. Ask mothers to freeze their breast milk in small single-feeding-size containers. Rotate frozen breast milk, using the oldest milk first, and keep it toward the back of the freezer where the temperature stays more uniformly cold. Throw out frozen breast milk after two weeks if it's kept in the freezing compartment of a refrigerator or after three to six months if it's kept solidly frozen in the freezer section of a refrigerator that has a separate freezer door. Once breast milk has thawed, do not refreeze it. Don't pour fresh or warm breast milk into a bottle of previously frozen breast milk. After a feeding, do not save or reuse leftover breast milk from the bottle. (For more information, go to the Centers for Disease Control and Prevention [CDC] Web site at www.cdc.gov.)

- Establish a labeling system so each baby gets his mother's milk; include the baby's name and the date and time the breast milk was expressed.

- Make sure the bottles of thawed or freshly expressed unfrozen breast milk are kept cold until they are consumed within five days.

- Keep hands, bottles, and equipment clean when handling breast milk.

- Thaw frozen breast milk in the refrigerator or under cold running water.

- If the mother prefers the breast milk to be fed warm, hold the bottle under warm running water or swirl it in a bowl of warm water just before giving it to the baby. Always make sure it doesn't get too hot. Do not heat bottles of milk on the stove or in a microwave, and do not store warmed breast milk or formula at room temperature. Shake heated milk so the temperature of the milk is evenly distributed.

- Always shake bottles of breast milk before feeding to overcome separation of fat that may have occurred during storage.

- Check whether your state or local public health office has regulations on storing and handling breast milk to keep it from spoiling.

- Provide breast-feeding information to parents (see further reading at the end of this chapter).

**PROMISING PRACTICE**

## Supporting the Breast-Feeding Mom

### WHAT WE SAW

Upon enrollment of each infant, the director and the teachers met with the parents to develop an individual nutrition plan for the child. Parents indicated their wishes for the nutritional health of their child, and a mutually agreeable communication system was developed. If the mother was breast-feeding and preferred privacy, she was provided with a screened-off area in the room. Teachers understood the importance of breast-feeding and of accommodating the mother's schedule.

**WHAT IT MEANS**

The teachers in this program understand there's a delicate balance in the way they communicate with parents, especially parents of very young children. Parents are often conflicted about going back to work after the birth of a child, and a respectful relationship with solid communication is important not only for the nutritional benefit of the infant but also for the emotional health of the parents. While meeting with the parents in person before the infant starts care may seem time-consuming, the development of a supportive caregiver-parent relationship is worth it in the long run. Meeting with parents has been known to prevent miscommunication and individual-care mishaps.

## Formula Feeding

While being supportive of breast-feeding, early childhood professionals must also respect and accommodate the needs of mothers and families who choose not to breast-feed their infants. For infants who are not breast-fed, iron-fortified infant formula is the only acceptable alternative to breast milk (American Academy of Pediatrics 2005). Iron-fortified formula may be fed as a supplement to breast milk in some circumstances, especially for older infants when breast-feeding is well-established. Some parents believe iron in formula causes stomachaches or constipation, but research has not confirmed this.

Caregivers who participate in the United States Department of Agriculture's (USDA) Child and Adult Care Food Program (CACFP) should be aware that iron-fortified infant formula is a required component of the meal pattern for babies who are not breast-fed (see appendix 2). Breast milk or iron-fortified infant formula is the only milk that should be fed to babies for their whole first year of life. Unmodified cow's milk, evaporated or condensed milk, goat's milk, soy milk, rice milk, almond milk, and nondairy creamers are *not* acceptable substitutes for breast milk because they do not have the proper balance of nutrients.

Standard rules for storage and pre-feeding preparation of formula are similar to the rules presented earlier in this chapter for breast milk:

- Always label bottles with the baby's name and the date and time it was prepared.

- Keep bottles of formula in the refrigerator until feeding time, and use refrigerated bottles within forty-eight hours.

- Throw away unused formula that is left in the bottle after each feeding.

- Warm a chilled bottle of formula immediately before the feeding by holding it under warm running water or swirling the bottle in a bowl of hot water. Shake the bottle and make sure the liquid inside is not too hot.

- Do not warm formula on the stove or in a microwave oven, because it is difficult to prevent overheating by using these methods.

Ready-to-feed formula is convenient and sanitary but more expensive than concentrate or powdered formula. When handling powdered formula, be sure everything that touches the powder, including hands and utensils, is thoroughly clean. Whatever type of formula is used, carefully follow directions on the container, making sure the bottles and equipment are clean. Water used for mixing formula must be sanitary and come from a source approved by the local health department.

---

### ✓ PRACTICE TIP

**Is It Safe to Make Baby's Formula with Well Water?**

Water from private wells is not always safe for infants. For example, in many parts of the Midwest, about one in ten private wells has bacteria or high levels of nitrate. Nitrates keep a baby's blood from carrying enough oxygen, leading to *methemoglobinemia*. Babies with methemoglobinemia, frequently called "blue baby syndrome," actually turn a bluish color around their lips, cheeks, and fingernails.

Boiling water does not get rid of nitrates or other chemicals. If your early childhood program has a water well or if families have their own wells, call the local health department for advice. The health department can lend advice about testing for other contaminants, such as arsenic, pesticides, and lead. You can also call the Environmental Protection Agency's Safe Drinking Water Hotline at 800-426-4791 or visit their Web site www.epa.gov/safewater to find out how to get well water tested.

### Water

In the first six months of life, healthy babies get all the water for their daily needs from breast milk or formula, even when their environment is very warm. Unless a physician gives specific recommendations for extra water, do not feed water to babies, and do not dilute breast milk or formula with extra water. After six months, water may be given from a cup if the infant is thirsty.

## Older Infants

### Feedings Should Nurture as Well as Nourish

The amount of food a baby eats is ultimately up to her, based on her internal hunger. Babies have different reactions to hunger. As a general rule, you can tell a baby needs to be fed when she becomes restless, sucks on her fingers or fist, or cries. Some parents and caregivers try to stretch the time between feedings to establish a convenient schedule, but this is not recommended.

It is important to give babies enough formula or breast milk (and semisolid food for older babies) to satisfy their hunger. Even if they are "chubby," underfeeding or restricting food is not appropriate for infants. On the other hand, feeding should stop when the baby is full. Do not coax a child to finish a bottle or serving of food, even if it seems wasteful not to. Babies show you they are full by spitting out or pushing the nipple away, pursing their lips together, turning away, or refusing to suck.

Hold infants in a partially upright position during bottle feedings. Gently burp young infants when they pause after a few minutes of sucking. Older babies who can sit up may hold their own bottles while sitting in a high chair, but this is also a good time for them to learn to drink from a cup. To reduce the risk of choking, babies should not carry their bottles with them when they crawl or walk around. Additionally, babies should not have bottles with them when they are put down for a nap. A form of dental caries known as *baby bottle tooth decay* can occur when a baby routinely goes to sleep with a bottle of breast milk, formula, or sweet liquid. The sugar in these liquids causes bacteria to grow rapidly and produce acid that wears away the hard surface on a baby's new teeth.

## MISTAKEN PRACTICE

## Feeding as a Chore to Get Done

### WHAT WE SAW

The new child care facility was bright and cheerful. In the infant room, four babies (eight to twelve months old) were lined up in their highchairs, each with a small jar of applesauce and a spoon in front of them. The teacher went from one baby to the next, lifting the spoon to the baby's mouth and then quickly moving on to the next child.

### WHAT IT MEANS

No doubt this teacher saved lots of time by lining the children up and speeding through their feedings. But feeding is more than a task—it is a key time for interaction with each child. Long ago, research on babies in orphanages found that even when they were fed enough and they slept enough and they had all their other physical needs taken care of, babies would become developmentally delayed in their social-emotional abilities if they had no regular, emotionally satisfying interactions with a consistent caregiver.

### WHAT WOULD WORK BETTER

Even before he can talk, a baby wants to communicate and interact. Talk with the baby as you feed him. Provide the words for his experience. "Oh, I can see you really were hungry. You really like this applesauce, don't you? Uh-oh, some of it is sneaking out of the corner of your mouth!"

## Developmental Milestones

Around four to six months of age, most babies are ready to start eating from a spoon, though they still get the bulk of their nutrition from breast milk or formula. At this age, tongue and mouth reflexes stop pushing food out of their mouths, they can swallow substances that are thicker than milk, and their necks and backs are strong enough to allow them to sit with support.

As the baby is exposed to greater variety in the baby foods she consumes, you can gradually increase the texture of the food, from smooth to slightly chunky. Chapter 3 has more information on helping babies and young children develop their eating skills, including self-feeding.

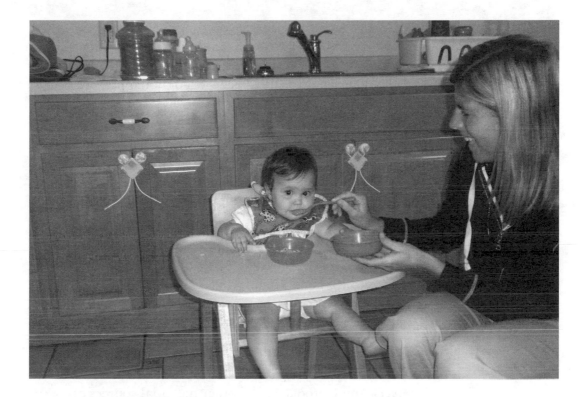

## Introducing Semisolid Foods

Ask parents for specific written instructions about which semisolid foods are being introduced and when. You may be asked to keep track of bowel movements during this period and to watch for possible signs of food allergies (rashes, diarrhea, vomiting). Traditionally, a mixture of breast milk or formula and iron-fortified, non-allergenic cereal is the baby's first semisolid food, followed by other infant cereals, vegetables, fruits, and then meats, poultry, and fish. For babies who have been exclusively breast-fed for the first six months, many experts recommend pureed meats as the first semisolid food, because they are high in iron and zinc. Egg yolk, yogurt, and small strips of cheese are considered okay for infants after about eight months of age.

Foods commonly associated with allergies (egg whites, peanuts, fish, and shellfish) are not recommended until the child is at least twelve months old, especially for babies with a history or high risk of food allergies. Honey should not be fed to infants under a year of age because it may contain spores that are more dangerous for babies than for older children (even pasteurized honey and baked foods that contain honey can have these spores). Raw (unpasteurized) cow's or goat's milk is *never* totally safe and should not be fed to children of any age, especially babies.

Other foods that may cause food poisoning include raw or under-cooked eggs, raw or undercooked meats, and improperly home-canned foods. Foods that have come in contact with saliva from the baby's fingers or spoon should be discarded. Homegrown or home-prepared beets, carrots, spinach, and greens may be high in nitrates and are not recommended for babies up to twelve months of age. (Commercial baby foods are tested to make sure the nitrate levels are low enough to be safe for babies.)

Keeping food and everything that touches food clean is important to prevent the spread of bacteria and viruses. Cleanliness in child care settings requires the following steps:

- frequent, thorough hand washing by children and staff and keeping tables, trays, plates, utensils, and equipment that touches food clean and sanitary;

- proper refrigeration (cold foods kept below forty degrees, freezers kept at or below zero) and keeping foods cold until they are ready to be cooked or served;

- storing and preparing foods in areas well away from dirty diapers, cleaning products, and other potential sources of contamination.

Appendix 4 has more information on food safety for early childhood settings. In addition, local and state licensing agencies and public health offices have recommendations or requirements for food preparation, service, storage, and general sanitation.

## Choking Hazards

As semisolid foods are introduced to babies, it is important to know that foods with certain shapes can become lodged in a baby's throat and block the airway, potentially choking the child. Particularly dangerous are, for example, whole grapes, hot dog sections, melon balls, cherry tomatoes, cubes of cheese, caramels, and other such semisoft foods. Hard pieces of food that can get stuck in the throat include hard candy, popcorn, snack chips, pretzels, and nuts. Large globs of peanut butter are also a potential choking hazard. To minimize choking, cut hard and semisoft foods into pieces that are smaller than the width of a child's throat, for example, thin shoestring strips, and have children sit at a supervised table while eating.

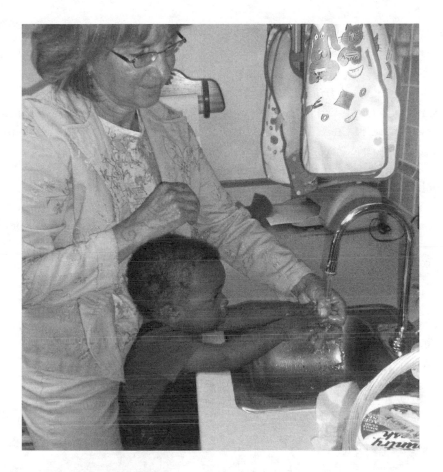

## ✓ PRACTICE TIP

### CPR Training

Most child care resource and referral agencies offer workshops on infant and child cardiopulmonary resuscitation (CPR), which is how to help a child who cannot breathe or whose heart has stopped beating. All staff members need to know how to handle such an emergency. Performing CPR can make a life-changing difference for a family. All child care providers need a current infant/child CPR certificate and first aid certificate from either the American Red Cross or the American Heart Association.

## Shun the Sweets, Snub the Salt

To help babies learn to like a variety of tastes, minimize the use of salt and sweeteners that tend to make everything taste similar. Cookies, candies, snack chips, fruit-flavored drinks, and soda pop have no place in an infant's diet. It is true that 100 percent fruit juice has much of the nutritional value of the fruit it came from, but it is lower in fiber. Fruit juice should be served in small amounts, because when babies drink too much juice, it displaces formula or breast milk and other nutritious foods to such a degree that their overall nutrition is affected. Fruit juice is not recommended before six months of age and should be limited to four to six ounces per day for children one to six years old (American Academy of Pediatrics Committee on Nutrition 2001). Diluting one part of 100 percent fruit juice with one to three parts of plain water is an option. Do not feed juices or other sweet liquids from the baby's bottle. Use a cup.

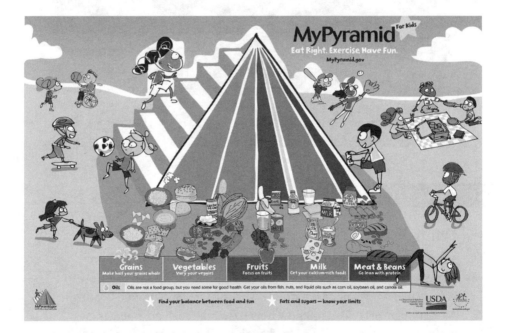

## ✓ PRACTICE TIP

### What Counts as "Added Sugar"?

The U. S. Department of Health and Human Services and the U.S. Department of Agriculture (2005) *Dietary Guidelines for Americans* and the USDA MyPyramid (U.S. Department of Agriculture 2009) define added sugars as sugars and syrups that are added to foods or beverages during processing or preparation. This does not include naturally occurring sugars, such as the sugar that's found in milk (lactose) or the sugars in whole fruits.

Most of the added sugars in American diets come from regular soft drinks; candy; cakes; cookies; pies; fruit drinks (such as fruit punch); ice cream; other sweetened, milk-based desserts; and sweet pastries. To find out if a food is high in added sugars, check the ingredient label for the following ingredients; they will be listed in order from high to low in terms of weight:

- brown sugar
- corn sweetener
- corn syrup
- dextrose
- fructose
- fruit- or cane-juice concentrates

- glucose
- high-fructose corn syrup
- honey
- invert sugar
- lactose
- maltose

- malt syrup
- molasses
- raw sugar
- sucrose
- sugar
- syrup

Some sweetened products are marketed as more natural because they seem more nutritious (those made with raw sugar, honey, or molasses, for example) or contain regular cane sugar (also called table sugar) instead of high-fructose corn syrup; however, when it comes to nutritional value, the differences between high-fructose corn syrup and regular sugar are negligible (American Dietetic Association 2008). Low-calorie sugar substitutes such as aspartame (Nutrasweet) or acesulfame K (Sunett) may help reduce consumption of added sugars in older children and adults, but parents and early childhood program professionals should avoid these substitutes when feeding young children. Although there is no direct evidence of their toxicity or physical harm, including added sugars in the diets of infants and toddlers may intensify youngsters' innate preferences for sweet tastes and make it more difficult to instill lifelong healthy eating habits.

**✓ PRACTICE TIP**

### What about Organic Foods?

Whether to purchase only organic foods is a question likely to invoke conflicting personal values and beliefs. Organic foods are grown without synthetic pesticides, growth hormones, antibiotics, genetic engineering, chemical fertilizers, or sewage sludge (Winter and Davis 2006). To qualify as organic, foods must come from farms that have been certified by the USDA. USDA inspectors verify that the foods were raised, processed, and distributed to meet official organic standards.

According to the AAP there is no evidence that foods labeled organic are any more nutritious or taste better than nonorganic foods. Similarly, the USDA does not claim that organically produced food is safer or healthier than food grown by conventional methods. Still, there are important reasons why early childhood programs may wish to emphasize organic foods in their meals and snacks:

• If anyone is likely to be sensitive to potential differences between organic and conventionally grown foods, it would be small children during rapid periods of growth and development.

• Organic foods tend to contain fewer pesticide residues than foods grown by conventional methods, though the differences are often poorly documented, inconsistent, or very small (Winter and Davis 2006). The Consumers Union (2008) has reported that organic apples, bell peppers, celery, cherries, imported grapes, nectarines, peaches, pears, potatoes, red raspberries, spinach, and strawberries are the fruits and vegetables most likely to be worth the extra expense.

As you weigh the pros and cons of organic foods for your program, consider the following factors:

• What do parents prefer? Some families may have political or philosophical reasons for preferring organic foods, or they may have a personal belief that they taste better.

• What do your local vendors provide?

• Are there differences in other aspects of quality (appearance, freshness, local sources)?

• What is the price differential?

Whether you decide to purchase all, some, or no organic foods for your program, it is vitally important to include a variety of fruits and vegetables and other healthy foods in the meals and snacks you provide young children. And all fresh produce, whether organic or not, needs thorough washing before it is eaten or prepared (go to the U.S. Food and Drug Administration [FDA] Web site at www.fda.gov for more information).

As you develop a policy for using conventionally produced or organically grown foods in your program, consult chapter 5, which provides information on establishing policies for early childhood programs.

## Infants and Toddlers Need Good Nutrition to Support Brain Development

While most brain development takes place before birth, young children's brains do continue to actively grow and develop during their first year and beyond. When infants and young children are chronically under-nourished, their brains are often smaller than normal, with fewer and less well-developed brain cells. Adequate nutrition in addition to mental stimulation and a nurturing environment is necessary for infants' and children's optimal intellectual, physical, and social development.

Some companies promote special "brain foods" that claim to maximize infants' and young children's IQs. Too often, such claims are exaggerated marketing ploys based on sketchy evidence. What we know for sure is that breast milk promotes optimal brain growth for infants up to six months of age. Around this age, infants' internal iron stores become depleted, and they need high-iron foods or supplements in addition to breast milk to get enough iron to keep their brains and bodies growing normally. Iron-fortified formula is recommended for non-breast-fed infants for similar reasons.

Other nutrients critical to supporting the normal brain growth of infants and young children include protein and fat. Studies show that a type of fat called *omega-3* (fat that is high in certain fatty acids called docosahexaenoic acid [DHA], eicosapentaenoic acid [EPA], and alpha-linolenic acid [ALA]) is important for early development of an infant's brain and eyes (National Institutes of Health and U.S. National Library of Medicine 2009). Omega-3 fats are found in fish oils, certain nuts, canola, soybeans, and flaxseed, and are added to many brands of baby foods and formulas.

Arachindonic acid (ARA) is another type of healthy fat (an omega-6 fatty acid) that may be important for early brain development. The current state of research on this subject is summarized in the following excerpt from a position statement of the American Dietetic Association and Dietitians of Canada (2007, 1606):

> Some studies have found benefits of including DHA and ARA in formulas for term infants, and no adverse effects of feeding marketed infant formula containing both ARA and DHA in amounts found in human milk are known. Because of possible benefits and lack of adverse effects, it is recommended that all infants who are not breastfed be fed a formula containing both ARA and DHA through at least the first year of corrected age.

## Feeding Toddlers and Older Children

Children keep growing rapidly after infancy, but their rate of growth in comparison to their size is slower than it was in the first year. Typically, children grow two to three inches taller and five or more pounds heavier each year after their first birthday (American Dietetic Association 2005). To maintain normal growth, nutritious meals and snacks should be offered every two to three hours.

Toddlers and preschoolers are at a critical stage for developing habits, preferences, and expectations regarding food and eating. In addition to providing age-appropriate portions (which are discussed in chapter 3) of healthy foods and beverages for meals and snacks, providers are urged to avoid the two extremes of being overly directive or overly permissive in guiding young children's eating (Birch and Fisher 1998). When adults are overly directive (for example, insisting that a child finish his vegetables or clean his plate), the result is likely to be that the child will later avoid the food the adult was trying to promote. On the other hand, allowing a child to have too much control over when or what she eats can also cause problems ranging from missed nutrition-education opportunities to a diet containing severely imbalanced quantities of sugar, salt, or solid fats (butter, stick margarine, shortening, lard) or foods heavily advertised to children.

A major study of preschool nutrition in the United States, the 2002 Feeding Infants and Toddlers Study (FITS) (Briefel et al. 2004), showed that most infants and toddlers consume too many calories and eat inappropriate foods as young as four to six months. Specifically, this study found that by age two, children's diets were too low in fruits and vegetables and too high in foods and beverages with added sugars, salty snacks, and juices. One of the most troubling findings was that french fries were the most commonly consumed vegetable by age two. Without counting french fries, more than one in four infants and toddlers had no vegetables on the day the parents answered the study questionnaire (Devaney and Fox 2008).

Appetites become fickle as infants become toddlers, and it becomes increasingly difficult to predict how much food a given child will consume at any particular meal or snack. Chapter 3 has more information on feeding children in a way that matches their physical, social, emotional, and intellectual development.

## "No, I Won't Eat That. I Want Something Else!"

Getting into a power struggle with a toddler is no fun for anyone. To avoid unnecessary power struggles, give children limited choices (see chapter 3). Choices let them feel some independence, but be sure the choices are good ones. For example, if a child refuses to eat the cucumber sticks you have prepared for snack, next time prepare both cucumber and zucchini sticks. Then give each child a choice between one or the other. Most children are happy to be able to choose. Avoid being too lenient with choices, or you may begin to feel like you've become a short-order cook.

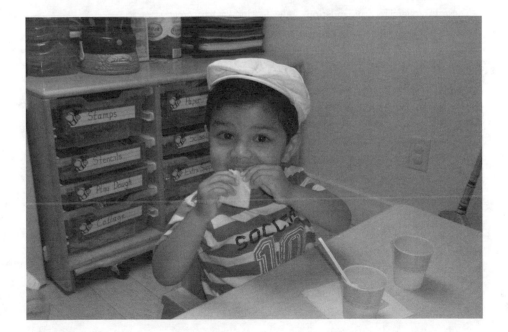

## Meal and Snack Planning Guidelines

In general, a child in a part-day program (four to seven hours) should receive food that provides at least one-third of his daily nutrition needs, whereas a child in a full-day program (eight hours or more) should receive foods that meet at least half to two-thirds of his daily nutrition needs (American Dietetic Association 2005). See calorie estimates provided in the table Daily Calorie Recommendations Based on Gender, Age, and Activity Level. Appendix 2 includes an example of an infant meal pattern and an example of a child meal pattern (pages 133–36). Appendix 3 shows an example of rotating Head Start menus that may be adapted for various early childhood programs.

### Daily Calorie Recommendations Based on Gender, Age, and Activity Level*

| Age | Fewer than 30 Minutes per Day of Exercise (Active Movement) | 30 to 60 Minutes per Day of Exercise | 60 or More Minutes per Day of Exercise |
|---|---|---|---|
| 2 | 1000 | 1000 | 1000 |
| 3 | 1200 | 1400 for boys 1200 for girls | 1400 |
| 4 | 1200 | 1400 | 1600 for boys 1400 for girls |
| 5 | 1200 | 1400 | 1600 |

\* These are general recommendations. Individual intakes vary greatly.

### ✓ PRACTICE TIP

**Tips for Providing Nutritious Meals**

• Buy most foods in their minimally processed forms (for example, frozen peach slices instead of peach-flavored fruit leather).

• Prepare a variety of foods from scratch. Include whole grains such as whole-wheat flour tortillas and whole-wheat bread.

• Read labels to choose items that are low in added sugars. For example, buy low-sugar yogurts instead of sugary ones with sprinkles.

• Use solid fats (butter, stick margarine, shortening, lard), salt, and sweets sparingly.

- Put apple butter or low-sugar fruit spreads on bread or toast instead of margarine or regular jams and jellies.

- Involve children in the daily preparation of their snacks or a portion of a meal by allowing them to perform safe, age-appropriate tasks several times a week. This experience gives children the opportunity to learn the basics of food preparation and cooking.

## ✓ PRACTICE TIP

### Tips for Saving Money When Buying Healthy Foods

The following recommendations are adapted from a University of Wisconsin-Extension press release on how to save money when buying healthy foods (Coleman and King-Curry 2008):

- Compare similar brands to find the best buy. If a store-brand cereal has the same ingredients and nutrients as a name brand (check the Nutrition Facts and ingredient labels) and tastes the same, the store brand will almost always be a better buy

- Dried beans, peas, and lentils are inexpensive and nutritious foods from the MyPyramid meat and beans food group.

- There is often a trade-off between convenience and price. Are you willing to grate and slice cheese? If so, blocks of cheese are usually cheaper, ounce per ounce.

- Many healthy snacks are also affordable. For example, a dish of yogurt, graham crackers and milk, and thin (shoestring) carrot strips with a homemade dip made from canned beans that are mashed and seasoned.

- If you have access to gardening space, grow some of your own vegetables.

- Watch for special seasonal prices and take advantage of them. For example, turkeys and fresh apples in the fall and grapefruit in the winter.

- When fresh vegetables and fruits are not in season, frozen and canned are usually a good substitute. They are typically just as nutritious, especially when you buy them plain. For example, buy frozen vegetables without sauce, and buy fruit canned in water or juice instead of in syrup.

> • When large quantities are cheaper and won't go to waste, buy the bigger package, divide into smaller amounts, and store for later use.
>
> For more information on this topic, see the Food Buying Guide for Child Nutrition Programs and other resources from the USDA Team Nutrition Program at http://teamnutrition.usda.gov (see the Resource Library link on the right of the page).

## Introducing New Foods

Learning to like new foods and new forms of familiar foods is important for two reasons: so the child learns to enjoy more foods, and so the child gains access to a wider variety of sources of nutrition. Many children become suspicious of new foods and refuse to even taste them. Caregivers should continue offering children a variety of nutritious foods without forcing the children to taste them. Adults can help by being good role models (Birch and Fisher 1998). It's okay if children politely take a new food out of their mouths; adults sometimes do this too. Since familiarity is the key to ultimate acceptance, don't be surprised if a child suddenly enjoys a food that she has refused to eat many times before. Offering new foods at the beginning of a meal when children are hungry may encourage more tasting.

**PROMISING PRACTICE**

### Contemplating Carrots

**WHAT WE SAW**

After reading the book *The Carrot Seed* by Ruth Krauss to a class of four-year-old Head Start children, the teacher divided the class into groups of six to eight children. The classroom assistant, cook, and teacher each worked with a small group. Each group leader placed several clean, fresh carrots of different sizes and shapes on the table for the children to examine. With direction, the children examined their carrots and described them (feel, shape, color, length, smell). The adults then asked, "I wonder if the carrot will taste the same and feel the same if it's cooked?" The adults cut a fresh, clean carrot into enough thin shoestring strips for each child in the group, and the teacher explained what she was doing as she cooked the carrot strips (in this case, using a steamer with appropriate safety precautions).

While the children waited for the carrots to cook, the teacher gave them crayons and paper and asked them to draw carrots, thinking not only about the carrots' colors, sizes, and shapes, but also about how they grow. As the children drew their carrot pictures, the teacher visited each child and said, "Tell me about your carrot." While holding a pencil, she said, "I'll write your story for you on your paper. What should I write?" She wrote one or two sentences dictated by the child. Then the small groups came together and the teacher read each child's story to the class as she showed the pictures. The class agreed to put the pictures together and make a book about carrots. They decided on a title, and the teacher stapled the pictures together. The children then tasted the cooked carrots and the thinly sliced fresh carrots and put a sticker under a raw carrot or cooked carrot picture to indicate which one they liked the best. Together the class counted how many children liked the cooked carrot most and how many children liked the raw carrots most. The cook explained she will serve both cooked and raw carrots during the coming weeks.

**WHAT IT MEANS**

One child may like thin strips of raw carrot, while another one may prefer cooked carrots. Sharing the wonder and being excited about trying new foods can have a profound influence on children and their attitudes toward trying and liking a variety of foods. By using the technique of *emergent curriculum* (as exemplified in the scenario above), teachers can involve children in decisions about trying new foods while guiding the experience with a sound knowledge of nutritional health and development.

## Physical Activity

Physical activity goes hand in hand with good nutrition in promoting healthy growth and development. Caregivers can help children be active by planning adequate time for supervised outdoor play every day when the weather permits. Aim to ensure that for every hour spent in a quiet activity like reading, ten minutes or more are spent in activities that involve active movement. Appendix 8 has suggestions for promoting physical activity in early childhood settings.

## Nutrition Education

Nutrition education should be integrated with other learning activities in a way that is age-appropriate, culturally sensitive, and coordinated with families. Younger children should be encouraged to learn about and enjoy a variety of healthy foods. As children get older, very basic concepts about the relationships between food and health can be introduced, along with an appreciation of where their food comes from. School gardens offer an excellent venue for children to participate in planting, tending, harvesting, and tasting vegetables and fruits. Children are more likely to try eating a food they grew, picked, or prepared themselves. They gain knowledge and familiarity with things by *acting* upon them.

Overall, the goals of nutrition education in early childhood are to

- form positive attitudes about food and eating;

- learn to accept a wide variety of foods;

- establish healthful eating habits early in life;

- learn to share and socialize at mealtime (in a group eating situation);

- be ready to continue learning while at child care.

---

**✓ PRACTICE TIP**

### Encouraging Children to Eat Healthy Foods

- Serve foods in a simple form. Very young children's taste buds tend to prefer food in a plain and simple form. Often young children prefer foods that are not mixed together—eating three cut-up fruits separately from a plate versus a mixed fruit salad, for example.

- Sit with children and eat the same foods they eat.

- Express enjoyment of foods as they are eaten.

- Talk about where a food comes from, its color, and how it promotes healthy bodies.

- Keep facial expressions, verbal responses, and body language pleasant and positive toward all healthy foods.

- Serve food in an attractive way. Children are often drawn to bright colors and foods that are eye appealing.

- Offer new foods several times each month. Repeat the new food in different forms and allow children time to get comfortable seeing and examining the food.

- Be patient and allow children opportunities to try new foods when they are ready.

- Serve food that is easy to handle and chew. This prevents unwanted frustration that may inhibit a child's ability to eat the food or to take interest in trying it.

- Involve children in growing, purchasing, preparing, and serving foods. This gives children a sense of ownership and commitment, which in turn encourages them to participate in consuming those foods.

- Read stories and plan classroom activities about specific healthy foods.

- Ask children who like the newly introduced foods to talk about why they like the food.

- Respond to a child's negative comments about a food in a positive manner.

- Serve "dessert" with the meal. Canned fruit (in water or juice rather than in heavy syrup) is an example. If your policy allows sweets, serve one small cookie with the rest of the meal to prevent the dessert from filling the child's stomach, if she chooses to eat it first.

## ✓ PRACTICE TIP

### Preschool Games and Activities for Nutrition Learning

- Play a guessing game with different foods (for example, apples, grapes, and peppers) in paper bags. Can the children guess the food item based on how it feels? The same game can be played with smells.

- Match pictures of two dishes that are made from the same food (whole-wheat bread in a sandwich and toast made from whole-wheat bread, for instance).

- Have a tasting party. The theme could match something you're doing in art or music.

• Read the book *Rabbit Food* by Susanna Gretz. Ask children to listen and to share their thoughts about whether John and Uncle Bunny are picky eaters. The overall theme is to encourage young children to try new foods, in this case celery, tomatoes, peas, mushrooms, and carrots (Michigan Team Nutrition 2002).

**PROMISING PRACTICE**

## Guided Learning

### WHAT WE SAW

A toddler classroom was having spaghetti for lunch. The teacher read the book *Daddy Makes the Best Spaghetti*, by Anna Grossnickle Hines, while some children sat on the rug and others listened as they played nearby. After the story, the teacher said that lots of different people make spaghetti and asked each child if anyone in their home makes spaghetti. Then the teacher told the children that they were going to have spaghetti for lunch and that she was going to show them some spaghetti before it was cooked. She showed the children the packaging the spaghetti came in and read the ingredients. Then she showed the children a few pieces of spaghetti. She talked about how the spaghetti was hard, long, and narrow and about how it breaks easily before it is cooked. She asked the children how they thought the spaghetti would change after it was cooked. One child said is would be "wiggly" and another child said it would be "soft." When it was time to wash hands to eat lunch, the children were very excited to see what the cooked spaghetti would be like, and they eagerly sat down to a conversation about the properties of spaghetti and about who in their homes cooks it. After lunch, as the children were settling into their cots for nap, the teacher asked the children to make their bodies look like spaghetti before and after it was cooked.

### WHAT IT MEANS

This teacher truly understands how linking children's experiences and literature with nutrition can provide a meaningful and rich learning experience for even young children. By beginning with a book about spaghetti, she gave information to children who may not have been exposed to spaghetti before. By drawing from the children's personal experiences, she helped some children further expand their knowledge of the preparation of spaghetti. Next, she broadened their experience by showing the box that holds the spaghetti and reading the ingredients. This exposed children to new vocabulary words and helped them gain a reference point for this product in their home or supermarket. By describing the texture of spaghetti before and after it was cooked, and linking that information to a movement activity, she cleverly integrated many concepts into the children's learning while encouraging gentle stretching. This teacher used a skillful guided-learning approach, which blends some instructional guidance with hands-on experiences for the children.

## ✓ PRACTICE TIP

### Ways to Promote Healthier Foods

• Serve nutritious foods in child-size portions or family style (as discussed in chapter 3). Let each child eat the amount he is hungry for that day. Power struggles often develop by insisting that children eat the most nutritious portions of a meal first and by regulating how much is required to be eaten before a child may have her dessert. Insisting that children eat their peas or drink their milk may turn mealtime into a negative experience and reinforce picky eating practices as the child grows older.

• Be a positive role model by sitting and eating the foods that are provided, especially new foods, as well as smiling while eating them. This is the best encouragement for children to try new foods.

• Talk about the food the children are eating. Describe its color, category, origin, and so on, to offer teacher-child interactions during mealtime.

• Without making a fuss, provide positive reinforcement for appropriate behavior such as tasting a new food or politely asking for seconds.

• Encourage parents to limit the amount of sweets provided at home. This gives children more opportunity to eat the healthy foods that meet their nutritional needs.

## Further Reading

### On Research

American Academy of Pediatrics. Committee on Nutrition. 2001 (reaffirmed in 2007). The use and misuse of fruit juice in pediatrics. *Pediatrics* 107 (5): 1210–13.

Auestad, Nancy, David T. Scott, Jeri S. Janowsky, Cynthia Jacobsen, Robin E. Carroll, Michael B. Montalto, Robin Halter, et al. 2003. Visual, cognitive, and language assessments at 39 months: A follow-up study of children fed formulas containing long-chain polyunsaturated fatty acids to 1 year of age. *Pediatrics* 112 (3): 177–83.

Birch, Leann L., and Jennifer O. Fisher. 1998. Development of eating behaviors among children and adolescents. *Pediatrics* 101 (3): 539–49.

Branscomb, K., and C. Goble. 2008. Infants and toddlers in group care: Feeding practices that foster emotional health. *Young Children* 63 (6): 28–33.

Greer, Frank R., Michael Shannon, and the American Academy of Pediatrics Committees on Nutrition and Environmental Health. 2005. Clinical report: Infant methemoglobinemia; The role of dietary nitrate in food and water. *Pediatrics* 116 (3): 784–86.

National Institutes of Health and U.S. National Library of Medicine. 2009. Omega-3 fatty acids, fish oil, alpha-linolenic acid. MedlinePlus. www.nlm .nih.gov/medlineplus/druginfo/natural/patient-fishoil.html.

Winter, Carl K., and Sarah F. Davis. 2006. Scientific status summary: Organic foods. *Journal of Food Science* 71 (9): 117–24.

### On Practice

Buck, Matthew. 2007. A guide to developing a sustainable food purchasing policy. Farm to School. www.farmtoschool.org/publications.php?id=207.

This guide was written to help advocates and institutions institute or promote realistic and sustainable food purchasing policies. This guide and other resources on purchasing food from local farmers are available online at the Farm to School Web site.

Color Me Healthy: Preschoolers Moving and Eating Healthy. www.colorme healthy.com.

This resource kit was developed by a partnership headed by North Carolina Cooperative Extension. It is a comprehensive, well-researched, and thoroughly tested set of interactive learning materials that promote physical activity and healthy eating for four to five year olds. It uses a combination of sensory experiences (taste, touch, smell, sight, and sound) to teach young children in family child care, Head Start, and preschool programs about eating smart and moving more.

Family Village. www.familyvillage.wisc.edu.

The Family Village Web site lists thousands of online resources with information on more than 300 diseases and conditions. Topics include assistive technology, legal issues, adaptive education, and ideas for active play.

National Association for Sports and Physical Education (NASPE). www .aahperd.org/NASPE.

NASPE has published recommendations for structured and free play for infants, toddlers, and preschoolers in *Active Start: A Statement of Physical Activity Guidelines for Children Birth to Five Years.*

National Food Service Management Institute. *CARE Connection.* www .nfsmi.org.

These resources include suggestions for nutrition activities to do with children in child care settings and information to send home to families on feeding children healthy meals. NFSMI also publishes training materials, recipes, and a wealth of other resources on food and nutrition for providers in child care and school settings.

Roberts, Susan B., and Melvin B. Heyman. 2000. How to feed babies and toddlers in the 21st century. *Zero to Three* 21 (1): 24–28.

U.S. Department of Agriculture. Food and Nutrition Service. 2002. *Feeding infants: A guide for use in the child nutrition programs.* Team Nutrition. www.fns.usda.gov/tn/Resources/feeding_infants.html.

This guide was written in 2001 and was being revised when this book was written.

U.S. Department of Agriculture. Food and Nutrition Service. 2003. *Nibbles for health: Nutrition newsletters for parents of young children.* Team Nutrition. http://teamnutrition.usda.gov/Resources/nibbles.html.

This set of newsletters was developed for child care center staff and parents who have young children enrolled in child care centers. The newsletters come with a CD that offers child care center staff guidance on conducting discussions with parents in three "sharing sessions" and includes accompanying posters. The kit features dozens of reproducible newsletters staff can provide to parents to address many of the challenges they face. This and other Team Nutrition resources from the USDA are available at http://teamnutrition.usda.gov/childcare.html.

U.S. Department of Agriculture. MyPyramid for Preschoolers. www
.mypyramid.gov/preschoolers.

This is research-based information on how the Dietary Guidelines
for Americans pertain to children ages two to five. You can develop a
personalized food plan for your preschooler based on his or her age,
height, weight, and physical activity levels. You can also complete growth
charts to find out more about normal development in the preschool
years. Ideas for developing healthy eating habits, trying new foods,
playing actively every day, and following food safety rules are included,
along with sample meal patterns, kitchen activities for preschoolers, and
recommended sources for more information (see excerpts in appendix 5).

Wisconsin Department of Health Services. 2009. Ten steps to breastfeeding
friendly child care centers. http://dhs.wisconsin.gov/health/physicalactivity/
pdf_files/BreastfeedingFriendlyChildCareCenters.pdf.

This resource kit begins with a self-assessment tool and explains ten action
steps that support breast-feeding families in child care centers.

## Breast-Feeding Resources for Parents

American Academy of Family Physicians. 2000. *Breastfeeding: Hints to help
you get off to a good start.* FamilyDoctor.org. http://familydoctor.org/
online/famdocen/home/women/pregnancy/birth/019.printerview.html.

Berggren, Kirsten. 2006. *Working without weaning: A working mother's
guide to breastfeeding.* Austin, TX: Hale.

Mohrbacker, Nancy, and Kathleen Kendall-Tackett. 2005. *Breastfeeding
made simple: Seven natural laws for nursing mothers.* Oakland, CA: New
Harbinger.

National Institutes of Health. 2009. Breast-feeding. www.nichd.nih.gov/
health/topics/Breastfeeding.cfm.

Pryor, Gale, and Kathleen Huggins. 2007. *Nursing mother, working mother:
The essential guide to breastfeeding your baby before and after you return
to work.* Boston, MA: Harvard Common Press.

U.S. Department of Health and Human Services Office on Women's Health.
2009. Breastfeeding—Best for baby, best for mom. www.4woman.gov/
Breastfeeding.

## Children's Books

Gretz, Susanna. 1999. *Rabbit food*. Cambridge, MA: Candlewick Press.

Hines, Anna Grossnickle. 1988. *Daddy makes the best spaghetti*. San Anselmo, CA: Sandpiper.

Krauss, Ruth. 1993. *The carrot seed*. New York: HarperFestival.

---

## When Teachers Reflect

### At a Nutritional Crossroad, How Can We Map New Directions?

By establishing healthy eating habits and attitudes and providing good nutrition for healthy development, early childhood programs act as a driving influence to reverse the alarming increase in the rate of childhood obesity and related problems such as diabetes and tooth decay.

How can our early childhood programs act as a driving influence to reverse this trend?

- How do we work with families and nutritionists to improve the nutritional health of children?

- Does our professional development include discussions to promote knowledge, skills, and dispositions in regard to nutritional health? Many state early learning standards have performance standards for the nutritional health of children, and the National Association for the Education of Young Children (NAEYC) includes nutritional criteria in their accreditation standards (see chapter 5). Implementing these recommendations and standards is the key to success, along with a review of our own attitudes toward nutrition.

- Are we good role models? We may think children aren't watching or listening, but we know intrinsically they are. It is critical to teach young children to trust their bodies in the regulation of hunger and appetite.

- Do we have knowledge about what healthy, nutritious choices are?

- Are we familiar with age-appropriate child-size portions?

- Do we have the skills to put our knowledge into practice while maintaining a positive attitude?

# Letter to Families: Active Play

All children need to be active. Movement builds strong bodies and helps prevent problems associated with being overweight or being obese. You also may have noticed that physical activity helps children burn off extra energy when they're feeling restless or fidgety.

## Did You Know?

Young children love to move and develop skills. For example, throwing and catching a large, soft (Nerf) ball helps build your child's coordination. As your child's physical skills become stronger, so does the child's enjoyment of active play.

## Things You Can Do

- Be a role model. Play with your child rather than just watch your child play.

- Set limits on TV and screen time. TV and videos are not recommended for babies at all. For older children, two hours is more than enough time to spend watching TV or videos or playing video games in any one day.

- Check out facilities in your neighborhood. Parks, recreation departments, clubs, and neighborhood associations often sponsor team activities, sports, and outings to help local children have fun while being active.

- Teach your kids to do the dances that were popular when you were a teenager.

- Imitate your favorite wild animals. Visit the zoo or a library to learn how animals move, and then build a family guessing game (like charades) around imitating the ways these animals get around.

- List your own ideas: _____

**Bottom line:** *Be active and have fun as a family. It will help everyone be healthier!*

From *Rethinking Nutrition* by Susan Nitzke, Dave Riley, Ann Ramminger, and Georgine Jacobs, with Ellen Sullivan, © 2010.

Redleaf Press grants permission to photocopy this page for classroom use.

# 2

# Special Needs

## Observation: Adapting to Varying Needs

*Martha knows the children in her classroom of three-year-olds very well. She also has a working relationship with the parents, because her program believes in serving the families and not just the children. When it comes to food, she knows Barry is allergic to wheat, Molly's family does not eat meat, and all the children have particular likes and dislikes. Respecting food needs and family values while teaching all the children to eat a variety of nutritious foods can be a challenge. Today's lunch of bean-and-cheese quesadillas with salsa, matchstick carrots, and milk is acceptable to all the families, but a few children have never eaten quesadillas and are cautious in trying this new food. All the quesadillas are made with corn tortillas (not flour tortillas) and no meat so that Barry and Molly won't be singled out.*

### A Mindful Approach

If every child enjoyed the same foods and grew at the same rate, life might be a bit boring but so much easier for the early childhood teacher! Young children have their own unique and often unexplainable preferences for some foods and not others. Families may have strong ideas about what is or is not acceptable for their children to eat. And some young children, like Barry in the introductory observation, have health reasons for particular diets. Dietary considerations are further complicated by the issues of obesity, on one hand, and undernutrition, on the other.

In addition to understanding and following regulatory requirements, early childhood programs need to thoughtfully attend to individual dietary needs. Commonly requested adaptations to meet the food and nutrition needs of children in early childhood settings follow. Chapter 5 contains suggestions for developing and sharing your program's food and nutrition policies.

## Overweight and Obesity

For children ages two and older, overweight is defined as a body mass index (BMI) between the eighty-fifth and ninety-fifth percentiles, and obesity is indicated by a BMI at or above the ninety-fifth percentile. These cutoffs are based on historic data of children the same age and sex. Ideally, children's BMIs are measured and interpreted by their pediatricians using growth charts from the Centers for Disease Control and Prevention (CDC). The CDC also provides an online BMI calculator for children at http://apps.nccd.cdc.gov/dnpabmi.

The prevalence of obesity among two- to five-year-olds in the United States has more than doubled since the 1970s, so more than 12 percent of preschoolers are considered obese (National Center for Health Statistics 2006). Obesity is more pervasive in some racial or ethnic groups. A nationwide study of 8,550 four-year-olds in 2005 found that American Indians had the highest occurrence of child obesity (31 percent), followed by Hispanic (22 percent) and non-Hispanic black children (21 percent) and then non-Hispanic white and Asian children (16 percent and 13 percent, respectively) (Anderson and Whitaker 2009).

Obese children and adolescents are more likely to be obese as adults (Freedman et al. 2007; Whitaker et al. 1997; Serdula et al. 1993). For example, one study found 25 percent of obese adults had been overweight as children, and if being overweight began before eight years of age, obesity in adulthood was likely to be more severe (Freedman et al. 2001).

Obesity isn't just about a child's appearance. Obese children are more likely than other children to develop high blood pressure, high blood cholesterol, asthma, sleep apnea (breathing changes that cause oxygen levels to fall during sleep), type 2 diabetes, or hepatic steatosis (fatty liver; fats inside liver cells). Certain psychosocial problems, such as discrimination and low self-esteem, are more common in obese children. Children and adults most often become obese due to a combination of genetic, environmental, and behavioral factors.

Child care plays a role in the development of obesity in young children (Benjamin et al. 2009). Harvard researchers found that time spent in child care was associated with an increased waist size at one year of age and BMI at three years of age, although the reasons why are not clear.

The strongest association of a child care arrangement (care in the family's home, at a center, or at someone else's home) to being overweight or obese was found to be care in someone else's home. What aspect of care in someone else's home was important for this outcome is not apparent; however, the findings imply that child care feeding practices can make a difference in children's likelihood of becoming overweight or obese during the early childhood years.

The most common causes of obesity in early childhood settings are

- serving overly large portions of foods and beverages;

- allowing frequent consumption of juice and high-calorie snacks;

- routinely serving fruit-flavored drinks, sodas, and other beverages containing added sugars;

- frequently serving meals and snacks dominated by highly processed foods (which generally have added fats and sugars) instead of basic, nutrient-rich foods;

- failing to provide sufficient opportunities and encouragement for physical activity and allowing children to spend too much time being sedentary (for example, watching television).

MISTAKEN PRACTICE

## Overreliance on Prepackaged, Calorie-Rich Snacks

### WHY THIS IS NOT SOUND NUTRITIONAL PRACTICE

Many prepackaged commercial products (processed foods) contain high amounts of added sugar, solid fats, and calories. While such foods may satiate hunger, they are not quality sources of nutrients needed for children's health.

### WHY WE SEE THIS MISTAKEN PRACTICE

Providers who work with children often have to be Jacks or Jills of all trades. Their trade work may include preparing snacks, cleaning up after snacktime, and being ready for the next activity. Also, foods easy to prepare and serve help providers meet the needs of hungry and sometimes impatient children.

## WHAT WOULD WORK BETTER

Many fruits and vegetables can be prepared ahead of time into child-size servings that are then ready to serve when it is snacktime. Oranges, cucumbers, green peppers, and zucchini are all easy to slice and store to later serve with a dip of yogurt or hummus. Grapes are super easy, as long as you cut them to reduce the likelihood of young children choking on them. Sliced apples can also be prepared ahead of time with a sprinkle of lemon juice to prevent browning. Cheese, healthy crackers, and fruit-based blender drinks (smoothies) are other options for providing healthy and yummy snacks.

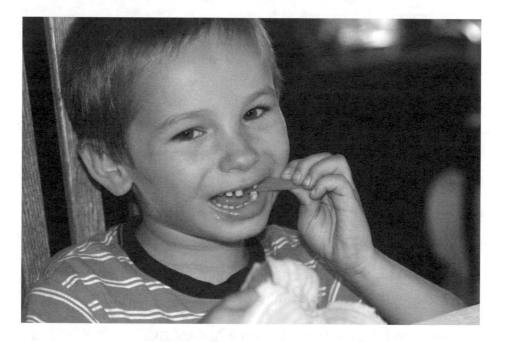

### ✓ PRACTICE TIP

#### Good Nutrition for All

All children, overweight or not, need proper nutrition. Therefore, as explained in chapter 1, the following practices are encouraged to promote health (and avoid contributing to children's overweight or obesity risks) for all early childhood settings (American Dietetic Association 2005):

• Emphasize nutrient-rich foods (vegetables, fruits, and whole-grain products) and limit consumption of foods that have added sugar and solid fat (often referred to as "processed foods") for meals and snacks.

- Serve low-fat or non-fat milk with meals for children ages two and older (whole milk is recommended for one-year-olds).

- Choose lean meats, poultry, fish, lentils, and beans for protein.

- Serve age-appropriate portions (allowing children to eat more if they're still hungry).

- Encourage children to drink water between meals when they are thirsty.

- Limit sugar-sweetened beverages.

- Work with a committee of nutrition-conscious parents to develop a list of acceptable birthday treats children may share at child care. Nix the cupcakes and sugary store-bought cookies. Your list may include items such as fruit cups, fruit smoothies, and frozen fruit juice pops. Some child care programs have a policy that treats supplied by parents must be store-bought and in original, unopened packaging. If this is the case, your committee's list may be limited in scope but will be just as helpful to parents. Child-safe trinkets, stickers, or art supplies (crayons and paper, for example) can replace food items as treats for a special occasion.

## Exercise

As children grow, their motor skills and coordination improve. Whenever the weather cooperates, children should be given at least sixty minutes of play outdoors a day, half of which may be during their time in care. Teachers and caregivers should engage children in fun and motivating physical activities. It isn't enough to take the children outdoors—some planning and organization really help (Sallis 2000). Appendix 8 provides suggestions for enjoyable ways to promote active play both indoors and out.

**PROMISING PRACTICE**

## Helping an Overweight Child Become More Active

### WHAT WE SAW

When the teachers got together and talked about which outdoor equipment each child preferred to use, they were surprised when they realized that no one had ever seen Joe on the slide, swings, or any of the climbing equipment.

## WHAT IT MEANS

Joe was overweight, and the teachers wondered if he was avoiding physical activity that was difficult for him. Joe's reasons for not using playground equipment may or may not have had anything to do with his weight. He might have been afraid of the height of a slide, or maybe in the past he had been hurt on playground equipment. Whatever the reasons, the teachers wanted to help Joe take part in using outdoor equipment and break a "vicious cycle" that may have ensued of avoiding exercise, becoming overweight, and enjoying exercise less and less.

## WHAT HAPPENED NEXT

The teachers made a plan to help Joe become more physically skilled and active. At the end of each day, while waiting for Joe's mother to pick him up, teacher Dave would work one-on-one with him for five or ten minutes. Dave used behavioral shaping, which means he helped Joe take the smallest possible steps toward improved physical ability and activity level. On the first day, Dave only asked Joe to step onto the first step of the slide, and Dave held Joe around the waist as they went up and down that step together. On the second day, Dave released Joe's waist for a few seconds before helping him down from the first step. It took nearly a month before Joe could independently climb to the top of the slide.

These steps may seem like ridiculously small accomplishments, but they demonstrate the keys to behavioral shaping: 1) never ask more of the child than he is currently capable of, and 2) as the child masters each new ability, push him a tiny bit further the next time. The hardest part for many teachers is finding a "first step" that is easy enough to ensure the child's initial success. Because Joe succeeded in each day's challenge, he soon looked forward to the time with teacher Dave, and his confidence increased as quickly as his ability and desire to take part in active playtime on the outdoor equipment did.

## Frequently Asked Questions

*Question 1: At what age are videos and TV appropriate for young children?*

Answer: The American Academy of Pediatrics recommends eliminating TV and videos for children under age two and limiting use of TV and videos to two hours per day for all other youngsters. The problem with TV and videos isn't only all the food commercials, but also that the time spent is "sedentary," displacing children's energy from more active and creative activities.

*Question 2: Is it okay to watch TV in bad weather?*

Answer: When the weather is bad and you need to keep children entertained indoors, the TV can be a handy tool. But rather than playing a movie or passive video, try showing videos of child-appropriate yoga, Tai Chi movements, or other activities the children can act out along with the video.

*Question 3: Are weight-loss diets recommended for young children who are overweight or obese?*

Answer: Young children who are overweight or obese should not be restricted to the point of going hungry, and they should never be forced to exercise in ways that feel like punishment. While these tactics may help restrict weight gain in the short run, more often than not they lead to feelings of deprivation and confusion that may result in unhealthy overeating and sedentary behavior in the long run. Instead, nutrient-rich foods and beverages that have less added sugars and solid fats than other foods and frequent opportunities for active movement throughout the day should be provided to *all* children in your program, not just children who are in the higher BMI categories.

## Failure to Thrive and Undernutrition

Children who are failing to thrive are growing too slowly. Generally, their weight or height or their rate of weight and height gain is significantly below that of other children who are their age and sex. Failure to thrive can be caused by medical problems, such as cystic fibrosis or premature birth, or by factors in the environment, such as child abuse and neglect or household food insecurity due to poverty. Treatment for children who fail to thrive usually requires an individualized plan incorporating medical, social, and nutritional interventions.

Parents of a child who is failing to grow properly should be consulted in establishing an appropriate feeding plan that can be implemented in the early childhood program as well as the child's home. Avoid the temptation to coax the child to eat high-calorie foods when she doesn't want to. Pressuring children who fail to thrive or are undernourished to eat more than they are hungry for or find appealing risks overriding the child's innate sense of hunger or satiety, as does forcing obese children to stop eating when they are still hungry. Ideally, the family's physician or a qualified dietitian should guide decisions about eating and help you and the parents monitor the child's progress.

If the family cannot afford medical care or does not have a primary physician, a local community health or family service agency should be able to help. In addition, food programs, such as the Special Supplemental Nutrition Program for Women, Infants, and Children (WIC), may be able to provide nutritious food and nutrition counseling.

Be careful to distinguish between failure to thrive and the seemingly sudden reductions in appetite that are common after the child's first year of relatively rapid growth. Erratic eating is not usually cause for concern unless the child's rate of growth is affected, which would be evident on the child's growth chart. Low weight or height are not enough to show failure to thrive but might indicate the need to take a closer look at the child. If a child was in the lowest 5 percent for weight or height as a baby and is still at the same level a year or more later, the child is probably growing normally at his own individual pace.

Appetite fluctuations can be exaggerated when young children establish their independence or bid for extra attention by refusing to eat. This can be challenging and frustrating for parents and early childhood professionals. In these cases, the best strategy is to avoid criticism and coaxing and, instead, focus attention on positive behaviors, such as when the child uses a serving spoon properly or helps another child find his napkin, and let periods of fussiness pass on their own.

---

**✓ PRACTICE TIP**

### Responding to Failure to Thrive

What should you do if you suspect a child is failing to thrive? Ask your local public health department (search online using your city or county name, state, and "public health department"). One option is to provide a free health screening to all the children in your program (to avoid singling out the child or his family), with a special focus on the child. Your job is to refer to health experts, not to make a diagnosis yourself.

Develop a directory of community support services for families with economic predicaments, health challenges, or other special circumstances and make it available to any family demonstrating a need. Your local Head Start program should be a primary resource. Head Start provides government-assisted meals and nutritional support for low income families with young children, as well as educational programs for early childhood.

## Diabetes

Diabetes is a group of diseases marked by high levels of glucose (blood sugar). Diabetes results from defects in the way insulin is produced by specialized cells in the pancreas and problems with insulin's ability to interact with cells as it circulates throughout the body. There are many kinds of diabetes, of which the most common are types 1 and 2. Children with type 1 diabetes are likely to be thin and have trouble maintaining a healthy weight without daily injections of insulin or other medications. Type 2 diabetes is associated with being overweight or obese. Type 2 diabetes is more and more common in older children, but it is still rarely seen in early childhood programs.

Meals and snacks for children with type 1 diabetes are usually planned according to carbohydrate counting methods and may use an insulin and carbohydrate ratio. Children who use this method take a prescribed amount of insulin for a certain amount of carbohydrates consumed. Ratios will vary from child to child and are prescribed by the child's physician. One example of an insulin and carbohydrate ratio would be 1 unit of insulin for every 15 grams of carbohydrates eaten. Proteins and fats should be consumed in moderation because these can over time help stabilize blood glucose levels.

Preschool children with diabetes need snacks to provide adequate calories and nutrients for growth. There is no need to provide special diabetic diet foods—all foods can be included, but it may be necessary to monitor the amount of food consumed and adjust insulin doses accordingly. Avoid using food as a reward. Plan ahead for special occasions, such as field trips. Ask families to provide specific instructions on how to monitor their child's needs if blood sugar levels get too low or too high. For example, parents may provide an easily swallowed carbohydrate supplement (for example, apple juice) and train the teachers to administer it if their child becomes sluggish or lethargic, both common signs of low blood sugar.

## Iron, Fluoride, and Lead

Iron deficiency anemia is one of the most common nutrition problems of childhood, especially during the first year or so when children grow rapidly. Severe iron deficiency can delay a child's mental and motor development, and in some cases a child's behavior and ability to learn are affected. This is why children are routinely checked for anemia during regular doctor visits, and it is the reason for using iron-fortified infant formulas for babies who are not breast-fed. Early childhood profession-als are not in a position to diagnose iron deficiency, but you can and should work with parents to make sure iron-rich foods (meats, fish, beans, fortified cereals) are offered at mealtimes. Iron supplements and other supplement pills should be kept out of children's reach, as excess intake of iron can be toxic.

Fluoride is another mineral frequently lacking in children's diets, es-pecially if they live in areas where the water is low in fluoride (American Dietetic Association 2005). Check with your community's water author-ity to see if your location or the neighborhoods served by your program are getting water with adequate fluoride (for example, between 0.7 and 1.2 ppm). If the fluoride is not adequate, families should be advised to ask their doctors about fluoride supplements to strengthen teeth and pre-vent tooth decay.

Many buildings constructed before 1978 have lead-based paint. If your facility was built before 1978, have it tested for lead (ask your pub-lic health department). Children who have been exposed to too much lead may suffer behavior or learning problems, so it is important that lead poisoning be detected early and treated properly. Blood tests are the only reliable indicator of lead poisoning.

## Food Allergies and Intolerances

Food allergies are common among young children, but not as common as some parents and caregivers think: about four percent of children under the age of eighteen have some kind of food allergy (Branum and Lukacs 2008). Children with food allergies are more than twice as likely as other children to have asthma or other allergies in addition to their food sensitivities.

The foods most likely to cause allergies in children are eggs, milk, peanuts, shrimp or shellfish, soy, tree nuts, and wheat. Many children outgrow food allergies as they get older, but allergies to peanuts, tree nuts, and shellfish are likely to be lifelong. Allergic reactions include tin-gling sensations or swelling around the mouth and lips; rashes or hives; gastrointestinal disturbances, including vomiting, cramps, diarrhea, or difficulty swallowing; nasal discharge or congestion; and wheezing or shortness of breath. In the most severe cases, allergies can interfere with breathing or cause a severe drop in blood pressure. Whether they are mi-nor or severe, food allergy symptoms usually occur within minutes after eating. They can be scary for both the child and you.

Make sure your program has up-to-date policies on handling and preventing allergic reactions (see chapter 5). For example, if a child in your care experiences a severe allergic reaction, she may need an immediate injection of epinephrine (a shot from an auto-injection device such as EpiPen or Twinject) to ward off anaphylaxis, an uncommon but serious whole-body allergic reaction that can be fatal (National Institutes of Health and U.S. National Library of Medicine 2009). If a family knows a child has a serious allergy, they may ask the early childhood program to keep an EpiPen, for example, handy and be ready to use it. If you do administer epinephrine to a child, notify the parents and have the child sent immediately to an emergency or urgent care center for medical evaluation and possibly further treatment.

## Food Intolerances

Food intolerances are similar to food allergies, but they do not involve the immune system. Lactose intolerance is the most common form of food intolerance, and it is especially prevalent among older adults from certain ethnic or racial groups. People with lactose intolerance experience gas, bloating, abdominal cramps, or diarrhea after drinking a glass or more of milk or similar amounts of lactose from other foods. Other than a temporary form of lactose intolerance had by children or adults with intestinal infections or diseases, lactose intolerance is not common in young children and is rarely encountered in early childhood programs.

---

### ✓ PRACTICE TIP

**Think of Your Class as a Family**

When planning how you will adjust meals and snacktimes to the needs of a child with any allergy-related diet restrictions, be sure to check with your child care licensing or local health department. Some state child care licensing regulations might require a physician authorization to address food intolerances and sensitivities. When a food allergy or intolerance diet fits your food policies and doesn't overly limit nutritious food choices for other children (see chapter 5), you will often find it easier to change the diet of the entire class than to have a separate diet and eating schedule for one child. Many families use this approach. If one member of the family can't eat a certain type of food, everyone else shares the dietary restriction to a reasonable extent. This makes meal preparation much easier, and you don't have to worry about an ingredient (shellfish or peanuts, for example) finding its way onto the plate of a person who will be harmed by it. And another reason to prepare the same food for everyone is that doing so provides some real social support for the person on the diet. The family—or your child care program—is saying, "We will not treat you differently. We are all in this together."

**PROMISING PRACTICE**

## A "Cool Cooking Experiences" Book

### WHAT WE SAW

The teacher in a two-year-old classroom wanted to do more cooking with the children, but had two children who were allergic to peanut butter and nuts. Many of the recipes he had used with children in the past called for peanut butter and nuts, so he called his local Extension office and the child care program advisers at his state Department of Education to get some new ideas. He also sent a newsletter home to families describing his desire to do more cooking with the children while being cognizant of allergies, nutritional health, and the introduction of new foods. Once he received feedback from families and nutrition program materials, he posted possible recipes on a family bulletin board and asked parents to add comments about the recipes. After he received feedback, he worked on his lesson plans to incorporate these cooking experiences and invited parents to join him and the children in implementing them. They even put together a "cool cooking experiences" book that families treasured for many years to come.

### WHAT IT MEANS

Nutritional considerations in early education are just as much a part of the curriculum as other areas of development, such as physical, cognitive, social, and language development. Experiences with food are inherently social, and by involving families, this teacher was providing opportunities for them to contribute to his curriculum design and to also get some great nutritional ideas to try at home with their children. By consulting an expert on allergies, this teacher recognized that he has expertise in child development and curriculum design but could benefit from the consultation of a health professional.

## Colic

Babies who have frequent episodes of uncontrollable crying are said to be colicky. This condition is especially common between six weeks and four months of age. The cause of colic is unknown; however, it appears to be associated with abdominal pain. Helping the baby burp more frequently or changing the time of feedings may help. The common belief that colic is a sign of a food allergy is probably inaccurate, but the baby's doctor may recommend a change in formula or in the breast-feeding mother's diet in case it might help. At present, colic is a condition that cannot be reliably prevented and must simply be lived with, although most children quickly grow out of it.

---

**✓ PRACTICE TIP**

**Mom's Familiar Scent Can Be Soothing to an Infant**

Did you know that the sense of smell is extremely powerful in infants and young children? When caring for an infant who has special needs or cries more, consider asking the mother to bring in an article of clothing that has her smell on it, such as a lightly worn T-shirt. Often infants will soothe easier when they can smell their mother's scent. While this will not cure colic, it is one way to respond to the sensory needs of young children.

---

## ADHD

Children with attention-deficit/hyperactivity disorder (ADHD) may be overly hyperactive, impulsive, inattentive, or all three. The causes of ADHD are not understood. Possible causes and risk factors include genetic (inherited) factors; brain injury; exposure to toxic substances, such as lead; prenatal exposure to alcohol and tobacco; premature birth; or low birth weight (see CDC information on ADHD at www.cdc.gov/ncbddd/adhd).

Impulse control, frustration tolerance, reflective problem solving, orientation toward the future, and delayed gratification are needed for all children and are especially important for children with ADHD (see chapter 3 on learning self-regulation in the first book in this series, *Social and Emotional Development: Connecting Science and Practice in Early Childhood Settings*). Reducing distractions, setting consistent limits, and providing positive attention can also help reduce behavioral and attention problems. The child's doctor may prescribe medication for older children with ADHD.

Although research has failed to pinpoint direct links between ADHD and nutrition, popular belief supports that there are. Sugar, synthetic sweeteners, food colors, and other additives are commonly blamed for ADHD. Although the value of nutrition treatments for ADHD is controversial at best, it is important to respect family requests and concerns about food within the limits and principles of your program's policies. Of the possible nutrition interventions, elimination of food dyes and increasing foods that are high in omega-3 fatty acids (fatty fish, walnuts, canola oil, flax) are most likely to help reduce symptoms in some children with ADHD.

## Vegetarian Diets

Total vegetarians (vegans) eat mainly grains, vegetables, fruits, legumes, seeds, and nuts. Generally, they do not eat meat, poultry, fish, seafood, eggs, dairy, or products made from animal sources. The vegan form is one of many subtypes of vegetarianism; subtypes depend on whether a vegetarian eats specific foods of animal origin such as dairy products, eggs, fish, or poultry. As a rule, well-planned vegetarian diets are nutritionally adequate and may provide health benefits in the prevention and treatment of certain diseases (American Dietetic Association 2009).

Iron-fortified commercial soy- or milk-based infant formulas are the only acceptable substitutes for breast milk for vegetarian infants for the first twelve months after birth. After their first birthdays, vegetarian children often drink fortified soy milk in place of cow's milk. Like cow's milk, soy milk should be full fat for one-year-olds.

The recommendations for introducing solid foods are the same for all babies (see chapter 1). Dried beans, soy products (tofu, tempeh, veggie burgers), other legumes (lentils, split peas), and nut butters are good protein sources from the MyPyramid meat and beans food group for vegetarians (American Dietetic Association 2009). Fish, eggs, milk, cottage cheese, and yogurt are also good protein sources that are acceptable to many vegetarians.

Expert advice from a knowledgeable physician or registered dietitian (RD) is strongly advised for vegan children, especially if there is any concern the child is not growing normally or he is not eating a variety of plant foods. The more restrictive the vegetarian diet, the more it's important that the child's food choices are carefully planned to assure adequate nutrition, especially for calcium, iron, zinc, vitamin B-12, and vitamin D. Food and nutrition experts at your state Department of Education or your child care resource and referral agency (CCR&R) may be able to suggest resources and provide advice on healthy vegan options, especially if they coordinate a federal food program.

## Disabilities and Chronic Diseases

Dietary changes are often required for children with disabilities or chronic diseases. Specific medical advice for these conditions is beyond the scope of this book, and it is important to work closely with the child's family and health care providers to understand accommodations that may be necessary.

Check with your state Department of Health or Education to identify programs that can provide assistance to families of children with disabilities and chronic diseases. The program for Children with Special Health Care Needs (CSHCN) provides a combination of benefits, such as case management, diagnosis, and treatment services. In addition, the Early Intervention program (EI) provides services to reduce developmental delay in babies and young children. These and other services are available in part because of "Section 504" which refers to a section of the Rehabilitation Act of 1973. Section 504 is a civil rights law that guarantees certain services and accommodations to individuals with disabilities, including ADHD.

### ✓ PRACTICE TIP

**Post a List of Special Dietary Needs**

With more emphasis on including children with disabilities in natural and the least restrictive environments, early childhood professionals can be important partners with families and early intervention personnel. Keep in mind that all children have varying needs; some children may have greater needs than others. When a parent asks if you can accommodate their child with special feeding techniques, such as using a feeding tube or adaptive equipment, keep an open mind. Each child deserves your thoughtful and caring attention to his or her nutritional needs.

Keep a list of dietary needs for children in your care. Post it in an accessible but confidential area, such as the inside of a food cabinet. Make sure all care providers, including teacher substitutes and cooks, know how to locate and use this information.

## Further Reading

### On Research

Benjamin, Sara E., Sheryl L. Rifas-Shiman, Elsie M. Taveras, Jess Haines, Jonathan Finkelstein, Ken Kleinman, and Matthew W. Gillman. 2009. Early child care and adiposity at ages 1 and 3 years. *Pediatrics* 124 (2): 555–62.

### On Practice

American Diabetes Association. 2008. Position statement: Diabetes care in the school and day care setting. *Diabetes Care* 31 (Supplement 1): S79–S86.

Family Village. www.familyvillage.wisc.edu.

Howell, Ensley. 2003. Diabetes fact sheet for child nutrition professionals. National Food Service Management Institute. www.nfsmi.org/documentLibraryFiles/PDF/20080908023024.pdf.

Kaczmarek, Louise A. 2007. A team approach: Supporting families of children with disabilities in inclusive programs. In *Spotlight on young children and families*, 28–36. Washington, DC: National Association for the Education of Young Children.

National Institute of Mental Health. Attention deficit hyperactivity disorder (ADHD). www.nimh.nih.gov/health/publications/adhd/summary.shtml.

National Resource Center on AD/HD. Ask a question about AD/HD: Section 504. www.help4adhd.org/en/education/rights/504.

Riley, David, Robert R. San Juan, Joan Klinkner, and Ann Ramminger. 2008. *Social and emotional development: Connecting science and practice in early childhood settings*. St. Paul, MN: Redleaf Press.

Roberts, Susan B., and Melvin B. Heyman, with Lisa Tracy. 1999. *Feeding your child for lifelong health*. New York: Bantam Books.

### Recommended Web Sites

Centers for Disease Control and Prevention. 2009. Childhood overweight and obesity. www.cdc.gov/obesity/childhood/index.html.

The CDC has a Web page that summarizes health issues and recommendations to address the problem of child obesity.

The Food Allergy and Anaphylaxis Network. www.foodallergy.org.

> The Food Allergy and Anaphylaxis Network promotes allergy awareness, education, advocacy, and research. The Web site includes fact sheets, recipes, and other resources. Parents of children with food allergies can connect at www.kidswithfoodallergies.org/index.html.

MyPyramid. U.S. Department of Agriculture. www.mypyramid.gov.

> MyPyramid has advice on vegetarian diets in the "tips and resources" section: www.mypyramid.gov/tips_resources/vegetarian_diets.html.

National Food Service Management Institute. www.nfsmi.org.

> NFSMI is a government-sponsored service with reliable advice on feeding children with special needs. A 2009 fact sheet on identifying food allergy symptoms is available online at www.nfsmi.org/documentLibraryFiles/PDF/20090210035621.pdf.

Nutrition and Physical Activity Self Assessment for Child Care program. University of North Carolina at Chapel Hill. www.unc.edu/~mwwhite/napsacc/index.html.

> Researchers at the University of North Carolina at Chapel Hill have been developing an instrument for self-assessment of physical activity and nutrition policies and practices in child care settings. The NAP SACC program had been pilot tested and was in the latter stages of a formal evaluation when this book went to print.

U.S. Department of Agriculture. National Agricultural Library. www.nal.usda.gov.

> The Food and Nutrition Information Center has a bibliography of resources on vegetarian diets.

The Vegetarian Resource Group. www.vrg.org.

> The "vegetarian family" section of the Vegetarian Resource Group's Web site has a wealth of resources on vegetarian diets for children and adults, including recommended books for young children.

Women, Infants, and Children (WIC). U.S. Department of Agriculture Food and Nutrition Service. www.fns.usda.gov/wic.

> WIC benefits are provided by the U.S. Department of Agriculture via state and local agencies. Breast-feeding and other postpartum women and children up to age five are eligible for WIC benefits if they are from low-income households and meet the nutritional need requirements. WIC benefits include supplemental foods, health care referrals, and nutrition education.

## When Teachers Reflect

### Thinking Ahead

Fear of the unknown tends to create anxiety. Gathering information and talking to others helps to ease fears, create understanding, and lead to professional growth. In order to understand the needs of families who have children with special needs, it is helpful to learn more about disabilities and the resources that are available for everyone, including the child, families, and early childhood professionals. Visit Family Village at www.familyvillage.wisc.edu to find disability-related resources. Click on the Family Resources icon to learn more about a topic of your choice. Report back to staff members at your next meeting, and share information in family newsletters, if appropriate. Some possible disabilities topics to explore are the following:

- What resources are available in your state?

- What are resources for child care?

- What is the Child Care Inclusion Challenge Project?

- What are resources for grandparents?

## When Teachers Reflect

### From Principles to Action

Children are individuals and have varying eating patterns and preferences. Teachers sometimes have the same standards for children as they have for themselves. If you do not like broccoli, you may not encourage children to eat it or you may through inadvertent actions indicate to children that it is an undesirable food. If you are not allergic to a food, you may forget about a child's food allergy. Other issues such as obesity or failure to thrive may bring forth unjustified assumptions about the child or family. Consider the following questions:

- How might your food preferences affect how you interact with children?

- Can you be a good role model if the children see you drinking soda?

- What safeguards can you put in place to ensure children are not exposed to foods they are allergic to?

- How can you in your daily routine and interactions be sensitive to the needs of children who are overweight or obese and children who are not overweight or obese?

# Letter to Families: Did You Know?

Young children love to demonstrate their independence by deciding what and how much they eat. Children with special dietary needs are not different. If children are pushed to eat certain foods, they often become less willing to try new foods. Involving your child in meal preparation and giving him or her appropriate choices will help your child learn there is more to meals than grabbing something quick and easy to eat.

## Things You Can Do

- Try serving a food in different ways: cooked, steamed, raw, or with melted cheese.

- Be a role model. Eat fresh fruits and vegetables as snacks. Have them ready as finger foods for kids.

- Limit sweets for the entire household. Save sweet desserts for special events (birthdays, holidays, awards or achievements, important guests, or sleepovers). Make desserts with nutrition in mind (such as homemade oatmeal cookies or pudding, or fruit-and-cheese trays).

- Introduce new foods in small servings or as a finger food.

- Don't overcook vegetables. Keep them slightly crisp, not mushy.

- Keep in mind that your child will be more likely to try new foods that look and smell good.

- Make nutritious food and beverage choices the most convenient ones. Instead of chips and soda pop, stock the refrigerator and cupboards with fruit cups; clean, cut vegetables; yogurt; cheese; low-salt nuts (for children over five years); whole-grain crackers and breads; low-fat milk; canned

From *Rethinking Nutrition* by Susan Nitzke, Dave Riley, Ann Ramminger, and Georgine Jacobs, with Ellen Sullivan, © 2010.

Redleaf Press grants permission to photocopy this page for classroom use.

tuna; and low-sodium, low-fat lunch meat (sliced chicken or turkey breast, for example).

- Plan regular times for meals and snacks rather than allowing your child to "graze" at will.

- Involve your child in the meal preparation process. Most children love to crack eggs, stir mixtures, knead dough, and measure with measuring cups.

- Buy a children's cookbook or borrow one from the library. Schedule time on weekends when you can help your child mix up whole-grain pancakes, or make grilled cheese sandwiches on whole-grain bread. Make sure the recipes are interesting and tasty but not loaded with sugar or solid fats.

- Use the Internet to look up kid-tested nutritious recipes. Together, you and your child can build a recipe book. Print out your child's favorite recipes and collect them in a binder. Encourage your child to draw pictures of the steps in the recipe, so he can read it.

- Develop your own recipes by supplementing ingredients that meet your child's preferences and health needs.

- Whenever it is practical, prepare meals and snacks from basic ingredients. For example, make your own chicken salad for sandwiches and pop popcorn on the stove in a covered pan with a little canola or other vegetable oil and minimal salt.

- Teach your child a new cooking skill each week. Techniques like separating eggs, peeling potatoes, and the proper way to measure flour can add to a child's confidence.

- Host a neighborhood nutritional food party with your child. Have each child bring a simple recipe with the ingredients, and take turns demonstrating how to prepare the recipe. Then everyone gets to taste each recipe.

From *Rethinking Nutrition* by Susan Nitzke, Dave Riley, Ann Ramminger, and Georgine Jacobs, with Ellen Sullivan, © 2010.

Redleaf Press grants permission to photocopy this page for classroom use.

- Make a food alphabet book with your child. Cut out the letters of the alphabet and pictures of nutritious foods from magazines and newspaper ads. Add a new letter every day or week (A–applesauce, B–broccoli, and so on). As you add letters and food names, serve the food as a part of your evening meal.

- Have family meals as often as possible each week. Keep TV, books, cell phones, and headphones away from the meal table.

- Encourage family discussions at meals. Play the "High/Low" game: all family members tell the others the best and worst things that happened during their day.

- Allow your child to decide when she has eaten enough. Coaxing a child to eat a specific amount of food teaches her to ignore internal feelings of hunger or fullness.

- Don't praise children for cleaning their plates. A child may overeat in order to please an adult.

List your own ideas: _____

_____

_____

_____

_____

_____

**Bottom line:** *Eat healthy and cook together as a family. It will help everyone be healthier!*

From *Rethinking Nutrition* by Susan Nitzke, Dave Riley, Ann Ramminger, and Georgine Jacobs, with Ellen Sullivan, © 2010.

Redleaf Press grants permission to photocopy this page for classroom use.

# 3

## Eating and Feeding Behaviors Are Formed in the Context of Normative Development

### Observation: Zucchini for Lunch

*When all eight four-year-olds were seated, teacher Sylvia told them they could begin serving the food. The children each took one large spoonful of food from the serving bowls and passed the bowls around the table. Sylvia said, "Here is the zucchini we picked on our field trip. See how we cut it into little rounds? And now it's cooked. Who said they had eaten zucchini before?" Two children had. "And did you like it?" One of them said she liked zucchini, and the other wasn't so sure. "Well, I like it a lot," said Sylvia. "I eat it all kinds of ways, sometimes even raw on my salads." Several of the children at the table used their forks to take cautious nibbles at pieces of stir-fried zucchini.*

Healthy eating habits are an essential part of good nutrition. With healthy attitudes toward food and mealtime, children learn to try new foods, control the amount of food they eat, solve little problems that can occur at the table (like spills), and generally perceive mealtime as a pleasant experience. Adults should present and guide young children's mealtimes in the following ways.

### Infants

Setting a feeding schedule dictated almost exclusively by the infant's hunger is the first step toward making mealtime enjoyable for both the infant and the caring adult. Mealtime is a great opportunity for caregivers to make a personal connection with each infant. By smiling, making pleasant sounds, and talking gently to the infant while feeding him his bottle, the conscientious provider is reinforcing eating and helping the infant remain relaxed in order to safely consume his nourishment. Adults know that children learn language by hearing it spoken. Infants begin to understand words often months before they begin speaking. By talking to the infant and telling him what you are doing and giving him encouraging words, the infant hears the adult's soothing sounds. Additionally, he feels the gentle secure movements of his provider as he is held while being fed. These behaviors introduce feeding to the infant in a warm and nurturing way, so the child associates food with a pleasant experience.

When the infant is able to sit up with support and swallow soft, mushy food from a spoon (around four to six months), parents and early childhood professionals can help her learn to enjoy new flavors and master increasingly thick and chunky textures. Often an infant will watch the face of the person feeding her. Again, the way food is presented will influence how the infant responds. Before feeding the child, some providers will take a small amount from the infant's bowl with another spoon and taste it while the infant is watching. By smiling, making pleasant sounds, and stating how good it tastes, the provider is role-modeling appropriate behaviors while showing the infant the food is something good to eat. Older infants will be able to use their fingers to sample various foods in semisoft, bite-size portions, using their gums to chew. The provider should be sitting and eating some of the same foods with the infants while talking to them and smiling. An observant adult will notice the individual needs and emotions of the infants and respond in a supportive way with a calm, reassuring voice.

---

### ✓ PRACTICE TIP

**Eating Is a Social Time**

Infants watch the faces of adults very closely and often model the emotions they see. If you wrinkle up your nose and look uninterested (or disgusted) at a certain food, the infant will sometimes imitate your reaction. Every infant should be given a chance to try a new food with enthusiasm. Even if you don't like the smell, texture, or taste of the food, smile and talk to the infant about what he is eating, how it is grown, and how it helps him grow.

## One-Year-Olds

In the second year of life, babies are growing rapidly in size, strength, and muscle coordination. They have a strong internal drive to explore their environment, including putting items (food and non-food alike) in their mouths. During this period, you can help one-year-olds learn to like a variety of nutritious foods by

- serving lots of different foods;

- giving them many repeated opportunities to sample nutritious foods, even if they are rejected at first;

- making mealtimes relaxed and cheerful (so they will be more inclined to try new foods);

- being a positive role model;

- allowing them to eat with their fingers and slowly master the skills needed to hold their own child-size cups and eating utensils.

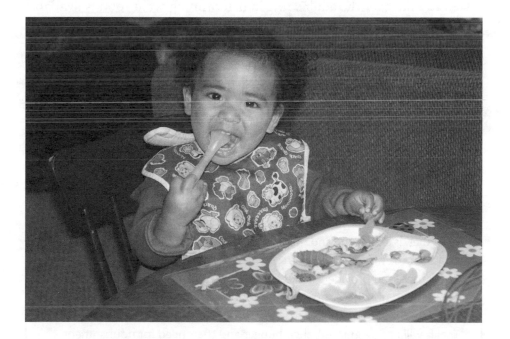

At this age, children quickly lose interest in eating when they are no longer hungry. By respecting these cues, the provider is helping children identify their natural body signs that they are full and stop eating. There is no benefit to the toddler's nutritional health if she is coaxed to finish the food on the plate. For many adults, this is an opportunity to correct a mistaken practice that they may have experienced as toddlers and young children. There's nothing to be gained by making a child feel guilty or ashamed if she leaves food on her plate because she feels full (see chapter 4 for more on this topic from a developmental perspective).

## Two-Year-Olds

As the overall rate of growth slows, the child's appetite may decrease, causing parents and caregivers to wonder if the child is eating enough to meet nutritional needs. Continue to allow toddlers to quit eating when they are full. As children are driven to explore limits and assert independence, they may refuse to eat foods they previously enjoyed. Toddlers may even refuse to eat anything served at mealtime. When this happens, calmly continue to offer nutritious foods and give the children an opportunity to eat at planned mealtimes and snacktimes. Children must decide for themselves how much to eat at any given time, but should not be allowed to take over the adult's role in determining what food is available or when. In other words, a child who refuses to eat anything at mealtime should not be given cookies or juice a few minutes after mealtime in an attempt to keep him from going hungry.

### ✓ PRACTICE TIP

**Offer Limited Food Choices**

Allowing children to determine their own dietary choices without any limits promotes poor diets and eating habits. The idea that children should eat different foods than adults, or that they get to choose their own diet, is a new one and not at all necessary or desirable. Letting a child choose his own diet is often one of the initial missteps parents and other food providers make, ultimately resulting in poor nutritional choices and possibly contributing to obesity. In contrast, once children learn that their requests for sweet or salty snacks in place of nutritious meals will not be granted, their hunger and their need for nourishment will prevail and they will eventually eat the nutritious meals put before them. Adult providers need to continue role modeling and reinforcing eating nutritious foods during mealtimes without forcing the issue.

Power struggles between provider and child over how much the child eats, or even whether the child eats a specific food or meal, are bound to end with unhappy and frustrated individuals. The key is to be patient and allow children to comply as they become ready.

## ✓ PRACTICE TIP

### Avoiding Power Struggles

Young children, especially toddlers, need help making healthy choices. So how do you handle a child who refuses to eat healthy foods? One way to help children develop both good nutrition habits and internal hunger control is to offer two healthy choices. Letting the child choose whichever food she prefers gives her some control and steers clear of the power struggle. If the child still refuses to eat, you can simply say these two choices are what is available now and the other choices will be offered at the next snack or meal. It is not recommended that adults require children to eat portions of their remaining lunch before they may have the snack being served. By doing so, the adult would be introducing a power struggle and teaching the toddler that meals will be frustrating experiences. As two-year-olds shift wildly between clingy dependence on adults and stubborn refusal of adult control over their behavior, begin addressing impulse control and self-regulation at mealtime, just as you do in other educational activities. (For more on offering appropriate choices, see chapter 3 in the first book in this series, *Social and Emotional Development: Connecting Science and Practice in Early Childhood Settings*.)

## Three- to Five-Year-Olds

Preschoolers' food preferences and eating patterns may continue to be erratic. Sometimes they will be so engaged in other activities they won't want to stop for a meal or snack. By this time, they probably have definite ideas of what they like and don't like to eat, based on their previous food experiences and observing the choices of adults and other children. That's why it is so important to serve as a positive role model. Advertising and marketing messages on TV and the Internet also have a strong influence on children's food preferences. Minimizing youngsters' exposure to commercial messages is very important at this age.

Preschoolers enjoy learning, and that should apply to food topics as well. This is a great time to read books about nutritious foods and cultural food patterns, as well as offer dramatic play experiences of eating nutritious meals. It is also a perfect age to show children how food is grown by having them help tend the vegetables in an early childhood program's garden or by visiting a local farm or orchard. Frequent classroom cooking experiences, in which children participate in preparing food, will also encourage preschoolers to try new foods and increase the probability that they will.

Pay close attention to the messages about food and eating in books during story time. Two researchers recently examined food messages in the most popular storybooks for young children and found that 38 percent of the 180 foods mentioned were "anytime" (most nutrient-rich) foods, 33 percent were "seldom" (least nutritious) foods, and the rest were "sometimes" foods that were in between in terms of nutritional value. Frequently mentioned *anytime* foods included apples and juices, while common *seldom* foods included cake, cookies, and ice cream. In the story lines, foods associated with "fun," such as at a party or celebration, were much more likely to be *seldom* than *anytime* foods (Byrne and Nitzke 2000). Stories that portray nutritious foods as fun should be chosen more frequently than cake-and-ice-cream books. See the end of this chapter for Web sites that list preschool-age books that encourage good nutrition and show fruits and vegetables as fun foods.

---

MISTAKEN PRACTICE

## Serving Only Familiar and Liked Foods

### WHAT WE SAW

A teacher of preschoolers complained to other staff that broccoli should just be taken off the menu because so many children don't eat it.

### WHY IT DOESN'T WORK

Children often need to try a new food a number of times—maybe eight to fifteen times—before they may decide that they like it. These trials include having the food prepared different ways to allow for the exploration of flavors and textures. If teachers simply assume children do not like something after they refuse it once or twice, they are giving up too soon. With a little patience, offering new foods in a variety of ways and with a positive (not pushy) attitude can make the difference between acceptance and rejection of specific vegetables and other healthy foods in a child's diet.

## WHY WE SEE THIS PRACTICE

Some food likes and dislikes are ingrained from the teacher's own childhood experiences. Maybe their parents made them eat foods they didn't like or maybe they have not been exposed to foods prepared in a variety of ways.

## WHAT WOULD WORK BETTER

Understanding that promoting nutritional health is as important as planning for other areas of development allows teachers to approach mealtime as an educational opportunity. Teachers can share with children the importance of sound nutritional choices and variety in their diets. Teachers' attitudes, words, and actions are all part of the educational process.

## All Ages

For all youngsters, adult supervision is essential during meals and snacks, but it can easily be taken too far. Studies show that children's food choices tend to get worse instead of better when they are coaxed, forced, or bribed to eat nutritious foods (Wardle et al. 2003). The strategies that have been shown to be effective in improving children's eating include

- minimizing the availability of, and attention given to, foods and beverages that are high in added sugars and solid fats (as discussed in chapter 1);

- offering age-appropriate portions (allowing children to ask for more if they're still hungry after a first serving);

- scheduling meals and snacks at regular intervals;

- providing positive social reinforcement for healthy eating;

- being a positive role model.

## De-emphasizing High-Fat, High-Sugar Foods and Beverages

Intuition and experience suggest that eating foods high in fat and sugars can lead to overeating, and research shows this is true. In a study at Pennsylvania State University, children ages three to five were served foods low in fat and sugar during breakfast, lunch, and afternoon snack. The researchers tracked everything the children ate for two weeks and found that overall calorie intakes were less during this period. The researchers explain their findings in terms of *caloric density*; that is, when children (or adults) are allowed to eat all they want of food that has a lot of calories packed into a small volume (calorically dense or calorie-rich foods like candy and chips), they may be more likely to overeat (Leahy, Birch, and Rolls 2008).

Eliminating sweetened beverages, both with and between meals, can help children avoid overeating (Keller et al. 2009). This was verified by a study that followed food and beverage intakes of girls when they were five years old and every other year through age fifteen. The study showed that greater consumption of sweetened beverages at age five was associated with a higher percentage of body fat, larger waist circumference, and higher body weight in later childhood and adolescence (Fiorito et al. 2009).

Many early childhood professionals realize sodas are not good for children's teeth, but they may not understand that fruit juice and fruit-flavored drinks are often major contributors of excess calories. In fact, data from national surveys show that juices and fruit-flavored drinks are the second and third most prevalent sources of calories in children's diets, exceeded only by the milk and breast milk or formula category (Fox et al. 2006).

---

### ✓ PRACTICE TIP

**Water**

Water is a very refreshing drink for both adults and children. Adding fresh cucumber, lemon, or lime slices gives water more taste and makes it special. If fresh cucumber, lemons, or limes are not available, additive-free lemon or lime juice is a good alternative.

## Portion Sizes

Serving age-appropriate portions to a group of children can be a challenge since children's hunger and appetite vary from day to day and from child to child. This is one reason family-style meals are encouraged in Head Start and other early childhood programs.

Experts recommend that caregivers serve small, child-size servings (usually two tablespoons to half a cup, depending on the type of food and the child's age) and give children the opportunity to ask for more if they are still hungry. Specific information about recommended portion sizes for children of various ages can be found in a 2008 practitioners' guide from the Nemours Foundation and the University of Delaware (see further reading).

## Scheduling

Timing and frequency of meals, snacks, and beverages help determine the quality and quantity of a child's food intake over the course of a day (Birch and Davison 2001; Fox et al. 2004). Snacks should not be allowed to crowd out meals as the main source of food. Similarly, sweetened beverages should not replace low-fat milk (or full-fat milk for one-year-olds) as the main beverage with meals.

If snacks are available within an hour of mealtime, the importance of the meal is compromised. Snacking just before a meal has the obvious drawback of reducing the child's hunger and interest in the food offered at mealtime. Allowing a child to snack soon after a meal sets up similar problems. The child may eat poorly at meals knowing he can fill up on snacks instead of the food served at mealtime. Many states recognize the importance of the frequency and quality of meals in regulations established for early childhood programs. Often early childhood professionals are required by law to provide a balanced meal or nutritious snack every two to three hours. Allowing young children to graze by having snack foods continuously available is not acceptable. In fact, food should not be served in intervals shorter than two hours or longer than three hours unless there is a special nutritional need. Of course, this does not apply to infants.

A program's snacktime may take various forms. For example, some programs have the classroom of children sit together when eating a snack.

Others may offer snacks as a choice over an interval of thirty to forty-five minutes. Regardless of the snack procedure used, children should be served a meal or snack at least every three hours.

Teachers should know each child's home situation and assist families in need with information on community programs that offer nutritional support. In some Head Start programs, for example, children are sent home with healthy snacks to share with other family members.

## Positive Reinforcement

Bribery (requiring a child to finish a specific food to earn dessert or a privilege like staying up late), begging, forcing, coaxing, and even bestowing excessive praise are all techniques that have been used by parents and teachers to get children to eat their vegetables. Unfortunately, even when they work in the short run, these strategies have been shown to have the opposite of the desired effect on the child's long-term food preferences. In other words, requiring a child to eat her broccoli before she can have a cookie is likely to increase the child's preference for cookies and decrease her preference for broccoli. Watching teachers and peers enjoy fresh broccoli and being able to taste the broccoli on their own terms are much more likely to help children taste and ultimately enjoy the flavor of broccoli.

The most effective forms of positive reinforcement tend to occur when a child does not expect a reward (no bribe has been offered) but is rewarded by the experience itself (good taste) or by a pleasurable social experience during the meal. When an adult makes too much of a child's good behavior, with obvious or extravagant praise, it often has the opposite of the intended effect, reducing the child's future preference for the food or activity (Greene and Lepper 1974).

Research has repeatedly shown that the most reliable way to build a child's taste preferences is through repeated exposure (Nicklas et al. 2001). Children often need to taste a food eight, ten, or even more times before they are willing to eat it. In addition to serving it often, you may be able to increase children's preference for a new food by serving it alongside a familiar and favored food (Pliner and Stallberg-White 1982). For example, the child's first exposure to a whole-wheat flour tortilla is likely to get a more favorable reaction if it is served as a quesadilla with melted low-fat mozzarella cheese.

Another way to heighten children's interest in, and familiarity with, nutritious foods is to give them a hand in growing, purchasing, or preparing it for a meal or snack. Gardens offer a great opportunity for children to appreciate where food comes from. Planting, tending, and harvesting a row of squash can't help but heighten the child's sense of investment in that vegetable's ultimate consumption. Appendix 6 lists several resources on gardening for early childhood programs.

**PROMISING PRACTICE**

## Growing Your Own Food

### WHAT WE OBSERVED

Three-year-old children poked a hole in the ground and buried bean seeds in the garden they helped cultivate. The children watered the bean garden and watched spouts come up several days later. By late summer, the children were given the opportunity to pick and wash a bean. More children preferred to eat their beans, rather than put them in a market basket to be sold to parents.

Children who were given the opportunity to water school garden vegetables and to pick vegetables of their choice, such as kale, spinach, lettuce, cherry tomatoes, peas, and beans rarely hesitated to try a new vegetable. Although not all children liked the taste of the vegetables, they often returned to try them again.

### WHAT IT MEANS

*Familiarity* is key to children's adoption of new foods. Repeated exposure to the taste of a new food (without pressure, coaxing, or bribery) is the best way to encourage ultimate adoption of the food. Growing the food and preparing it for a meal is an ideal way to create familiarity. These are great examples of *learning by doing*, the very best way to learn. Even adults are more likely to eat food they have grown and cooked themselves!

## Being a Role Model

Observational learning from role models is one of the main ways children learn many types of new behavior. Research has shown that observational learning also applies to what and how a child eats. When a parent, teacher, or respected adult sets a good example by enjoying the flavor of a nutritious food, the child's acceptance of that food is given a boost (Hobden and Pliner 1995).

PROMISING PRACTICE

## Modeling Nutritious Eating

### WHAT WE SAW

A teacher picked some peas from the garden and asked the two- to three-year-olds, "Who wants to eat a pea?" A few excited children put their hands out. The teacher then said, "I love the taste of peas, they're so juicy," and proceeded to eat a pea. She ate a few more peas as the children watched. She then again asked the group of twelve children who would like to try a pea. All but one of the children put up their hands.

### WHAT IT MEANS

This teacher not only models the behavior she wishes to encourage (eating peas), but also uses language to describe the experience favorably. By talking out loud, she makes sure the children understand the experience she is modeling. The early adopting children were also role models for the others. The second time she asks if anyone would like to eat a pea, most children could not resist the excitement of the other children waving their hands for a pea!

## Manners

As a teacher, you know young children are developing motor skills. Children observe the way family members and teachers eat and try to do the same, within the limits of their coordination and motor skills. As they progress beyond getting food from a bottle or being spoon-fed by an adult, older infants and toddlers eat mostly with their fingers. Two- and three-year-olds become slightly less messy and clumsy as they learn the skills needed to handle child-size utensils and cups. By the time they are ready for kindergarten, most children have mastered the basics of eating the way adults do, with diminishing rates of spills and messiness.

Just as children need practice to handle the equipment used at mealtime, they also need practice to learn and master the behaviors that are socially acceptable at mealtime. Those exact practices vary from culture to culture and by the formality of the setting, but the principles are the same. Ultimately, children need to learn to behave in ways that keep mealtimes pleasant for themselves and others at the table.

Setting age-appropriate limits, explaining expectations, serving as a positive role model, and responding to negative behavior by describing and reinforcing the more acceptable behavior help children learn to say "please," use a napkin, or take turns (see chapter 4).

---

**✓ PRACTICE TIP**

**Handling Messes and Spills**

None of us should ever be surprised when a child makes a mess or spills food. Even adults do this sometimes!

• Don't make a big deal out of it, and avoid making the child feel bad about it.

• Use a neutral, accepting, matter-of-fact tone to help the child solve the problem and get back to the task at hand (eating).

• Provide just enough help so the child can clean up his spill. You might remind the child where the sponge is or, if the child is very young, you might need to get a sponge and bucket and demonstrate how to clean up the mess. Learning to clean up a mess is a life skill, and this is a chance to learn it. Focus on the child's growing competence to perform the skill of cleaning up one's own messes.

---

## Family-Style Meals versus Teacher-Served or Family-Provided Meals

All early childhood program directors must decide on the procedures for and sources of meals served at their site. Considerations such as the facility's space and equipment, funds available, and nutritional goals affect how and what meals are served in each program. A family-style meal is one in which foods for the whole group are provided in serving bowls and the bowls are passed around the table, with the teacher and each child dishing up his or her own serving of food. Other mealtime styles include teacher-served and family-provided food. Teachers do not eat with the children in teacher-served meals. Another type of teacher-served meal may be delivered from an outside source and prepackaged as individual servings. A family-provided meal or snack is usually prepared for the child by her parents and eaten individually—it's not shared, and each child eats only what has been provided for her from home. Also, family-provided meals might be dished up by the teacher and set out for children to eat from their plates. In all these examples of teacher- or family-provided meals, the children have premeasured food served to them.

## Benefits of Family-Style Meals

- Children practice eye-hand coordination and self-help skills through serving themselves.

- Children develop the abilities to judge a serving amount and to make choices of food they believe they will eat.

- Children learn to share food, leaving some for their classmates.

- Children learn to eat what is served and experience a sense of inclusion and security that comes from a group eating the same foods together.

- Children are more likely to be exposed to new foods (and as a result try new foods) when meals are served family style. A four-state study showed that teachers discussed the food more with children in programs in which meals were served family style (Sigman-Grant et al. 2008).

- Teachers are more likely to serve as positive role models by trying new foods with the children during family-style meals.

- Families may prefer that the program prepare family-style meals for their nutritional value and convenience.

## Drawbacks of Family-Style Meals

- Allergies, food sensitivities, and the cultural practices of a few children may cause programs to exclude many nutritious foods from their menus.

- There is a greater risk of food waste with family-style meals. Children are prone to misjudging the amount of food they can actually eat. Children serving themselves often spill. In addition, most child care food regulations require served foods not consumed to be discarded.

- Children may sneeze or cough into the serving bowls or touch food in the serving bowls, exposing the food to germs and contamination.

- The cost to provide state-approved kitchen facilities and additional trained staff to prepare meals or to have catered freshly prepared meals may not be feasible for a program.

- If one child refuses to try a food and makes an issue about it, many other children will respond similarly.

- Families may have difficulty affording the program's planned meals. If a family-style meal program is optional, children not participating in it may feel excluded from the group.

## Benefits of Teacher-Served or Family-Provided Meals

- Families can control and monitor the amount and content of food their children eat when the food is prepared at home.

- There is less waste, and uneaten food can be sent home.

- Families are able to maintain special diets or culturally approved meals.

- Children often look forward to eating a lunch they know was prepared for them by a parent. It acts as a connection to their home and parents. Often parents will include encouraging notes to their children in the lunch bag sent from home.

- Programs may be able to lower the overall cost of child care when parents provide meals.

## Drawbacks of Teacher-Served or Family-Provided Meals

- Children may get less exposure to new and differently prepared foods.

- Children may have fewer opportunities to develop table skills and manners.

- Opportunities for teacher-led discussions about the food the children are eating may be more difficult and less frequent.

- Opportunities for experiencing a sense of community may be compromised as children eat different foods and do not share the same meal together.

- Families often send individual pre-packed lunches that lack variety and may not have the nutritional quality of meals provided by institutions that follow nutrition standards.

Some programs have found a way to use some of the benefits of both styles by serving school-prepared snacks family style and serving home-prepared meals. Occasional, special classroom meals delivered from restaurants or family invited potluck meals are ways to help offset the drawbacks of family-provided meals. Family potlucks provide the additional benefit of including parents or others in sharing the meal.

---

**✓ PRACTICE TIP**

**Encourage Autonomy without Wasting Food**

When children are encouraged to serve themselves, sometimes they put too much food on their plates. Perhaps their hunger really seems that large at the time, or maybe they just enjoy using the big serving spoon. Whatever the reason, the result is a lot of food going to waste because children simply cannot eat that much. How can teachers encourage autonomy without wasting good food? Use smaller serving spoons and have rules, such as only take two scoops the first time and if you are still hungry later you can have more. Also, cut sandwiches into fourths and fruit into smaller sections.

---

**✓ PRACTICE TIP**

**Partnering with Families**

If families do not have access to markets with high-quality, affordable produce, you may provide information on local sources for healthy foods. For example, low-income families with children under age five may be eligible for WIC benefits in the form of coupons or electronic debit-style cards that can be used at grocery stores and farmers' markets. Your local Extension or public health office may offer nutrition education programs, gardening classes, or referrals to assistance programs.

## Conclusion

The following advice from Ellyn Satter (2008), an internationally recognized authority on child feeding, sums up the information in this chapter: children need adults to be supportive and companionable, to show them what it means to grow up with respect toward food, and to give them opportunities to experiment and master.

## Further Reading

### On Research

Fox, Mary Kay, Kathleen Reidy, Timothy Novak, and Paula Ziegler. 2006. Sources of energy and nutrients in the diets of infants and toddlers. *Journal of the American Dietetic Association* 106 (1): 28–42.

Riley, Dave, Robert R. San Juan, Joan Klinkner, and Ann Ramminger. 2008. *Social and emotional development: Connecting science and practice in early childhood settings.* St. Paul, MN: Redleaf Press.

Roberts, Susan B., and Melvin B. Heyman, with Lisa Tracy. 1999. *Feeding your child for lifelong health.* New York: Bantam Books.

Wardle, J., M. L. Herrera, L. Cooke, and E. L. Gibson. 2003. Modifying children's food preferences: The effects of exposure and reward on acceptance of an unfamiliar vegetable. *European Journal of Clinical Nutrition* 57 (2): 341–48.

Zens, G. 2009. Wisconsin homegrown lunch: The arduous road to better school lunch. *Sustainable Times* 5:1–5.

### On Practice

Hendricks, Charlotte, and Paula Mydlensky. 2006. Family-style eating. In *Nutrition in childcare: The best of healthy childcare.* Healthy Child Publications. www.healthychild.net.

Nemours Foundation. 2008. Best practices for healthy eating: A guide to help children grow up healthy. http://static.nemours.org/www-filebox/nhps/childcare-kit.pdf.

Delaware's Child and Adult Care Food Program (CACFP) and the Nemours Health and Prevention Services developed this nutrition guide of best practices to help young children develop healthy eating habits early in life. In this booklet, you will find guidelines for healthy foods and portion sizes, rationale for the recommendations, and sample policies.

Nickols-Richardson, Sharon M., Danielle E. Parra, and Elena Serrano. 2009. Nourishing children with books. Virginia Cooperative Extension. www .pubs.ext.vt.edu/348/348-950/348-950.html.

This resource supports children's development of reading skills and promotes learning about food, nutrition, and physical activities that encourage healthy lifestyle choices. Appropriately selected books and follow-up activities can improve reading skills, enhance an interest in reading, and support good food and physical activity choices for children.

## Children's Books

The Michigan Team Nutrition program has created a list of books for preschoolers with positive messages about good foods, available at www .tn.fcs.msue.msu.edu/Michigan%20Team%20Nutrition%20Preschool%20 Booklist.pdf. Chapter 4 contains a list of recommended children's books on food, cooking, and gardening. One of our favorite examples is *The Carrot Seed*, first written by Ruth Krauss in 1945.

---

## When Teachers Reflect

### Differences in Families' Meal Table Expectations

Many young children have families that do not have regular routines, so children do not know when to expect their next meal or snack. Children may not sit at a table to eat at home and may not be expected to use basic table manners. Do you know children who might fit this description? How can you guide their behavior to fit in with the social expectations of the child care setting while maintaining their sense of self-esteem? What are realistic expectations of children for table manners at various ages? What are some positive ways to reinforce these manners?

## When Teachers Reflect

### Using Food in Art Projects

Should food be used in art projects? If helping adults grow, cook, or serve carrots, for example, boosts a child's interest in tasting those carrots, wouldn't making an art project with carrots have the same effect? Maybe, or maybe not. There is no research on whether playing with food in a non-meal context helps a child learn to like the flavor of that food. We suspect using carrots in an art project may increase the child's overall familiarity with carrots, but the potential for mixed associations may override the benefits. After all, if you're not supposed to eat other art materials (paint, paper, glue, and string), why should the carrots be different? Are the children getting plenty of other opportunities to experience nutritious foods using all their senses? How many cooking and meal preparation opportunities are available on a weekly basis? Cooking and meal preparation are appropriate activities for children to explore food with their senses. After all, isn't food intended to be eaten?

Using food for classroom projects can offend some families, especially if they have lived through hard financial or economic times or if they are currently threatened by hunger at home. In efforts to be sensitive to families, many preschool teachers do not use food for play or art. Others have made a compromise and will use foods in their non-edible state, such as dried beans and corn in sensory tables or uncooked noodles in art projects. Whatever the practice, it is important that early childhood programs develop a policy regarding the use of edibles in the classroom for purposes other than eating and publish it in their family handbook. More information on the topic of policies can be found in chapter 5.

# Letter to Families: Making Mealtimes Pleasant and Healthy

If mealtimes become unpleasant or a power struggle with children, then children are more likely to grow up with poor nutrition or eating problems. That's why, in addition to caring about your child's nutrition, our early childhood program also cares about *how* we feed and eat with the children.

- We encourage children to help us serve food and set the table.

- We use child-size tables, chairs, glasses, silverware, and serving utensils that young children can handle, so they learn more easily to do things for themselves.

- We eat together, family style, and make it a pleasant time with conversation.

- We help the children as they serve themselves a small amount of each food and pass the serving dishes to the next person at the table. Children may ask for seconds after everyone has had their first helping of the food.

- We allow children to leave food on their plates. Our job is to provide them nutritious and tasty foods, and their job is to eat according to their feelings of hunger rather than the amount on their plates.

- We never use food as a bribe, reward, or punishment.

- When children refuse to eat or make a fuss at mealtime, we quietly correct their behaviors. If the child is too tired or upset for a quiet correction, then it's time to end the meal rather than get into a difficult power struggle.

These methods work for us. If you wish to learn more about making mealtimes pleasant as well as nutritious, talk with us.

You may also read more about ways to promote good nutrition for your child in the "developing healthy eating habits" section of the MyPyramid for Preschoolers Web site www.mypyramid.gov/preschoolers/HealthyHabits/index.html.

From *Rethinking Nutrition* by Susan Nitzke, Dave Riley, Ann Ramminger, and Georgine Jacobs, with Ellen Sullivan, © 2010.

Redleaf Press grants permission to photocopy this page for classroom use.

# 4

# Food and Mealtime as a Context for Learning

## Observation: Lunchtime Learning

*"Spaghetti!" shouted Allisa. "I can't wait!"*

*"We have to wait until everyone is seated and everyone is served," replied Mario, repeating the rule the teacher has been reciting to her class of three-year old children since the fall.*

*Finally Deshawn sat down. Several of the children had been visibly sitting on their hands, successfully but impatiently waiting. "We may serve the lunch now," said teacher Emily in a quiet voice from her seat at the end of the table. The children began serving themselves from the bowls in the middle of the table and passing the platters of bread around. "Has everyone been served?" asked teacher Emily. "Yes, yes!" shouted the children. "All right then, bon appétit." The children began eating with gusto. For about twenty seconds, the only sounds were of eating. Then teacher Emily looked around and asked, "Who can tell me what spaghetti is made from?"*

Meals are important for their nutrition, but what happens during meals around the table is also important. In many studies, researchers have consistently found that responsive, well-organized, and well-regulated mealtimes predict better child outcomes in a wide variety of areas (Fiese and Schwartz 2008). Mealtimes seem perfectly designed for many kinds of children's learning, in large part because they are a consistently structured time that recurs every day (Larson 2008). Children can experience

the benefits of a group mealtime in their early childhood program regardless of whether they have this experience at home.

Mealtimes can have an impact on children learning

- social skills (such as sharing, impulse control, and self-
responsibility);

- intellectual skills (such as language and preliteracy abilities);

- knowledge of the natural world (science).

## Mealtimes

In many cultures, family mealtime is a highly organized group activity
that happens most days of the week. Mealtimes become ritualized; the
family goes through the same pattern of behaviors at the same time each
day, and most families have unwritten rules about how everyone should
act. Researchers call these ways of acting *normative expectations* or just
*norms*. A family might, for example, have the normative expectation that
no one will take seconds of a food until each person has been served, or
that children will stay at the table until they finish their meal and are ex-
cused, or that everyone will say something about what they did that day.

Norms for family mealtimes vary quite a bit from one culture to another and from family to family within cultures (Hall, Nagy, and Linn
1984). For example, conversations in Israel have been reported to focus
on some event from the past that everyone shared, while conversations in
the United States are more likely to tell people at the table about an event
they missed. Even in cultures with strict rules about formal, polite behavior at mealtime, there is considerable family talk (Blum-Kulka 1993).
There are interesting differences in how mealtime is shared in families
and cultures, and there are also interesting similarities.

Families of different cultures and income levels in the United States
tend to share the same understanding of what family mealtime should
be like: all members of the family are together, it lasts more than just a
few minutes, and everyone around the table contributes to pleasant conversation (Dickinson and Tabors 2001). Of course, some families have a
hard time succeeding in actually making a custom of family mealtime. A
parent's job or children's group activities can occur at times that conflict
with a family meal. Even the enticement of eating out or watching television shows while eating can interfere with families establishing patterns
of eating and conversing together.

An early childhood program that creates its own customs and rituals around group mealtime can offer many of the benefits of family mealtime for those children who do not experience it at home. Creating a well-organized day, in which the child knows what to expect next and what behavior is expected of him, is important for all young children, but is especially important for children who live in disorganized households or are going through changes in their lives. For example, research on children whose parents are divorcing has found that when strong household routines are maintained, such as family mealtimes, the children fare much better (Hetherington 1992). When family routines fall apart after a divorce, children are also likely to be disorderly. Similarly, a child who is going through any kind of stressful or unsettling period, such as the birth of a younger sibling or a change of residence, will be especially helped by well-established routines in the early childhood setting. Another example of this principle is the child who is new to the early childhood setting and who really begins to feel at home in the program when he or she learns the daily schedule and rhythms well enough to anticipate them. The regularity of a well-ordered group mealtime in the early childhood program adds the comfort of predictability and a sense of control to a child's life, while teaching children some of the common cultural norms around shared meals. Because research has confirmed that parents learn from their early care and education programs, parents visiting the program and observing the mealtime may also adopt the same custom of a family mealtime at home (Riley et al. 2008).

## Social Development around the Meal Table

Almost everything a child needs to learn about getting along with others can be taught around a meal table. In fact, the meal table is just about perfectly designed for social learning, since it is a group setting and activity that recurs each day at the same time, with well-defined roles and a common purpose. Learning how to share or take turns is easier at the meal table than at less frequent or well-patterned activities like sharing a favorite toy or taking turns using a glue stick. Helping children learn to share a glue stick is a great opportunity to teach them how to solve problems by sharing, but passing the food plate is even better because it takes place every day and because the pattern of sharing becomes a kind of habit or ritual.

## Problem Solving

One of the difficult and crucial *developmental tasks* of early childhood is learning how to solve conflicts with other children in competent and socially acceptable ways (in other words, without pushing or hitting). This is difficult for young children because of two conflicting trends that arise during the toddler years: 1) maturation pushes toddlers to exercise increasing *independence* and *autonomy* (this is why they like to say "no"), and 2) adults must exert *socialization pressure* on them, teaching them that they cannot always get their own way, that the needs of others are also important.

When frustrated, toddlers at first tend to simply strike at their source of frustration. When another child picks up their toy, they tend to grab it back, hit, or bite. Early childhood programs teach children more socially acceptable ways to respond to such daily frustrations, usually in the form of three behavioral skills: taking turns, sharing, and telling the other child how their behavior makes them feel.

The common rules of behavior at meal tables reflect social lessons that toddlers must eventually master. The idea that everyone gets one serving is an expression of the idea of sharing. Passing a serving platter around the table is an example of turn-taking. The inevitable disputes which arise from one child bumping another or one child taking another's cup of milk provide opportunities teachers need to instruct children to "use your words" (rather than your teeth or hands) to express displeasure with another person's actions. With most toddlers, saying "use your words" will not be enough, and you will need to teach them the exact words to use, such as "Tell Jaime, 'I don't like it when you bump into me.'" Given that an adult is always monitoring the meal table, mealtime recurs each day, and the rules of behavior are always the same and consistently enforced makes mealtime ideal for these basic lessons in social living.

## Behavioral Self-Regulation: Impulse Control

Behavioral self-regulation, or impulse control, includes both the ability to stop oneself from doing something and the ability to control the speed at which something is done. It may come as a surprise that young children first learn how to perform an action and only later learn to regulate that action. They learn to grasp an object, such as a cracker, and later learn to let go of it or to stop themselves from reaching for it. They learn to hold a small pitcher and tip it to pour milk (with a lot of patient trial and error), and later learn to tip the pitcher more slowly.

At age three, most children cannot successfully play Red Light, Green Light. They cannot stop themselves from going whenever any light comes on! But by age five, most children can go on green and stop on red. In similar fashion, three-year-olds cannot consistently draw a line slowly across a page. They seem to have only one speed at which they draw. They get better at regulating the speed of their drawing each year up through age six (Maccoby 1980).

As you can imagine, behaving well is very difficult for a toddler who does not yet have impulse control. When a toddler hears "don't touch the cookies," he gets the idea and image of a hand touching the cookies, and he will usually act on that idea immediately. It is always better to tell toddlers to do something else instead: "Help me get a paper napkin to put over the cookies, to keep them warm." The teaching and learning of self-regulation is one of the keys to good behavior. The most well-behaved children have internal control, so that adult control is less necessary. (For more on the development of self-regulation, see our earlier book in this series, *Social and Emotional Development: Connecting Science and Practice in Early Childhood Settings*.)

The meal table is full of opportunities to teach behavioral self-regulation. The observation at the beginning of this chapter describes such a program, in which the children have learned to wait until everyone is seated at the table before they begin serving the food. The teacher has even taught them that no one can begin eating until everyone has been served and she gives the signal, "bon appétit!" These are hard rules to learn and follow, but learning is much easier at the meal table than it is during most other parts of the day because the situation is repeated every day and the situation itself begins to reinforce the learning. Each child comes to expect and remember the rules as soon as they approach the table. The teacher can help children learn by modeling the correct behavior and describing it in words: "I'm really hungry, but I can wait until everyone is served."

---

✓ **PRACTICE TIP**

### Replace "Don't" with "Do"

When a child begins to misbehave at the meal table, the easiest and first thing most adults say is "Don't." Don't play with your food. Don't touch Miguel's food. Don't take any more carrots until everyone has some.

A better strategy for fostering impulse control is to phrase sentences to create positive images of a better behavior in the child's mind.

- Instead of "Don't play with your food," try rephrasing your request to "Sally, please use your fork to eat."

- Instead of "Don't touch Miguel's food," you could say, "Try to pick up your beans with your spoon."

- Instead of "Don't take any more carrots," you could advise, "Before you take any more, please pass the carrots so everyone gets some."

Monitor how often you say "don't" and force yourself to rephrase your directives in positive terms. Saying "don't" is not teaching, it only prohibits. In contrast, you are actually teaching when you tell a child how to do something right or competently. Instead of "Don't spill the milk," which teaches nothing, you could say, "Use your helper hand under the pitcher. That's it!"

## Cognitive Self-Regulation: Planning

Young children are impulsive not only in their actions but also in their thinking and decision making. Learning to think ahead and plan one's actions is a key ability for any future success. Researchers have found that children with a low ability to plan and organize their own actions tend to have more behavioral problems in elementary school (McClelland, Morrison, and Holmes 2000).

Children differ greatly in this ability, and early childhood teachers can help all children learn how to be more self-regulating. The following are some of the key methods a teacher can use.

FORESHADOW. Warning children that it is almost time to finish their activities, put things away, and clean up for lunch is an example of foreshadowing. When you help children think about what happens next and the order of things, it gives them time to prepare for the transition and a sense of control over events. "After we have finished lunch, we will need to clean the table before we can go outside."

MODEL A COURSE OF ACTION. Teachers can model out loud a planful approach to thinking, so the children can see how the teacher organizes her actions. "Let's see; before we can set the table for lunch, what do we need to do first? That's right, we need to wash our hands."

OFFER WELL-MATCHED TASKS. A toddler might not be able to plan all the things that need to be done before lunch can be served, but she can be given small parts to do, such as putting a plate in each place or a cup at each plate. As they gain in ability, you can give children a larger role in planning, by asking, for example, "What things do we need to put out for each person?" This is called *scaffolding*, which means providing the necessary support for a child's early attempts to master new skills and then withdrawing your support and asking more of the child as she's able to do more of the task unaided. By the end of the year, you might be able to assign two children to prepare the table, and they might be able to do the entire job themselves.

Because the meal table (or snack table) has a routine, it is an ideal setting for teaching children to anticipate and plan their future actions.

## Self-Regulation May Affect Future Obesity

Not only can young children learn self-regulation (impulse control and the ability to delay gratification) at the meal table, but their learning can also affect later eating behaviors and health.

Researchers found that some three-year-olds were able to avoid touching an exciting toy when left alone in a room with the toy for over a minute and fifteen seconds, whereas other three-year-olds could not resist touching the toy. This was a measure of impulse control. The researchers tested the same children at ages four and five for their ability to delay gratification. First the researchers had each child pick their favorite of three snacks (candy, crackers, or pretzels), and then the child was given the choice of eating a small stack of the snack right away or waiting for the researcher to return to the room before they could eat a larger stack of the same snack. Three-year-old children who were able to wait longer had a greater ability to delay gratification.

The results showed that preschoolers who scored lower on these tests of self-regulation gained weight more quickly over the next few years. This may seem surprising, because in the tests they chose to eat the *smaller* amount of snack immediately. But the key is that they were not able to delay their eating, because their impulse control and ability to delay gratification were low. By the time they were eleven or twelve years old they were significantly more likely to be overweight, even after controlling their initial weight (Francis and Susman 2009; Seeyave et al. 2009). Clearly, helping preschoolers develop their ability to self-regulate is a key part of helping them become adolescents who make wise choices about food and health and actually become more healthy.

MISTAKEN PRACTICE

## Pushing Children to Clean Their Plates

### WHAT WE SAW

A toddler teacher strongly believed that children should eat everything on their plate. Children were told it is wasteful not to eat everything and were forced to stay at the table until they had tried everything.

### WHY IT DOESN'T WORK

Insistence on finishing the food on one's plate may seem like a good way to teach children the value of food, but it may be ill-advised for a number of reasons: 1) children often resist this type of pressure, and needless power struggles may ensue, 2) a child's internal sense of fullness is more important than the amount of food on her plate as a determinant of how much she eats during a given meal, and 3) many experts believe repeated episodes of eating to please someone else may set up a pattern of overeating that may lead some children to overweight or obesity.

### WHY WE SEE THIS PRACTICE

It's normal to dislike seeing good food go to waste. This teacher may also have grown up being forced to eat everything on her plate and feel that it is shameful to throw food away. Children sometimes serve themselves too much food because it is so much fun to use the big serving spoon.

### WHAT WOULD WORK BETTER

Young children have small stomachs, uneven growth patterns, and appetites that normally vary greatly from day to day. Teachers should help them maintain their innate sense of food intake regulation based on their feelings of fullness. Experts recommend serving or offering age-appropriate, child-size portions of nutritious food (roughly a tablespoon for each year of the child's age) and giving children the option of asking for or serving themselves more if they're still hungry or leaving food on their plate if they choose not to eat it. This gives children appropriate choices of what to eat and lets them know it's okay to stop eating when they feel full. If children are allowed to serve themselves (usually a good idea), then teachers can place limits on the number of spoonfuls they can take at a time, so they do not give themselves too much food. When new or unfamiliar foods are rejected, offering the food several times (on different days and without pressure) and acting as a positive role model are likely to have more desirable outcomes than pressuring children to eat specific amounts of food.

## Practical Life Skills and Self-Responsibility

One of the founding influences on early education was the work of Maria Montessori (Roopnarine and Johnson 1993). For example, Montessori was the first (a century ago) to introduce child-size chairs and tables, small pitchers for pouring milk, and even small scissors for little hands. She produced these child-sized tools so that young children could do more things for themselves, taking more responsibility for their own doing and learning. One of her key domains of learning in the early childhood years was *practical life skills*, and the meal table is one of the key places for learning these skills.

In the same way that young children can pour their own milk if you show them how and provide child-size equipment, children can also learn to do many of the other chores related to mealtimes. For example, they can learn to

- clean the table before lunch;
- wash their hands before setting the table or eating;
- set the table with plates, cups, and utensils;
- carry serving bowls to the table;
- serve themselves;
- push in their chairs when leaving the table;
- take their plates and utensils to the kitchen for washing;
- clean the table after lunch.

You may have noticed that practical life skills are often chores that need doing. The toddler ages (beginning in the second year of life) are the very best time to start having children do things for themselves (like clearing their plate from the table) as well as do chores for the group (like setting the table). Children at this age love to copy the actions of adults, so doing a chore seems like fun to them, and they are proud of their increasing competence.

One study that assigned household chores to young children found that preschoolers felt a great sense of pride in being able to accomplish the chores. Their parents, who often were skeptical about their children

handling chores, were pleased with their children's enthusiasm and feelings of success (Wallinga and Sweaney 1985). If prompted to do so,
most parents with young children like to assign them chores, believing
it teaches responsibility, builds character, and creates a sense of family
unity (White and Brinkerhoff 1981). Parents are often surprised to see
their children doing chores in the early childhood program, and learn
from the program that they might ask for such help at home as well.

There is little research on the impact of practical life skills and chores
on toddlers and preschoolers, but one excellent study followed slightly
older boys into adulthood to see the effects of early responsibility. In this
forty-year longitudinal study of inner city boys, those who worked either at regular part-time jobs or had regular household chores grew into
adults who were happier and more competent than their peers (Felsman
and Vaillant 1987). This was true regardless of their level of intelligence
or their parents' education, income, or jobs. The researchers suggested
that work or chores may have fostered a sense of self-competence that
helped the boys develop resilience in managing future challenges.

## ✓ PRACTICE TIP

### Teaching Practical Life Skills

- Avoid trying to teach many skills at once: adopt them within the classroom
  one at a time.

- Foreshadow: tell the children in advance about the new responsibility they
  will have.

- Explain and demonstrate: show children how to do the chore, and explain
  what you are doing while you are doing it.

- Practice with feedback: have the children give it a try, provide feedback
  on how they are doing, and focus your attention mostly on what they are
  doing right.

- Provide supports: if you want children to wash the table before mealtime,
  then provide them with small buckets and sponges; if you want them
  to clear their plates and utensils after the meal, then provide a place to
  put them that's low enough for their reach. Make it easy for children to
  succeed.

- Give reminders: for many days you will need to patiently remind children of
  the need to do the chore and how it should be done.

## Intellectual Development around the Meal Table

Just as with social development, mealtime is well suited for teaching and learning many of the lessons of intellectual development. This is largely because preparing and eating meals is an activity, so children can learn through their own actions about something they care about (food!). The possibilities for language development, mathematics learning, and natural science knowledge (especially chemistry and biology) are especially visible in excellent early education programs.

### Language and Pre-literacy Development

The snack or meal table is a great place not only for good nutrition, but also for good conversation. Both the nutrition (as discussed in chapter 1) and the conversation are important for children's success in early education and later schooling.

In fact, researchers can predict the growth of young children's vocabularies by recording family conversations around the dinner table. Frequency of family mealtimes is associated with greater vocabulary growth and academic achievement (Beals and Snow 1994). A study that followed children and families for several years showed that the use of unusual words during mealtimes at age two predicted larger vocabularies at age five (Snow and Beals 2006). A larger vocabulary at age five is crucial because vocabulary size at entry to elementary school tends to predict later reading performance and school success (Morrison, Alberts, and Griffith 1997).

To enlarge their vocabularies (the number of words they recognize and can use), children need not just language stimulation but, more important, language *interaction*. They need an adult nearby who knows more words and who can engage the child in joint attention to the same topic, to label the child's experience and actions and engage her in back-and-forth conversation. A mealtime, when everyone is seated together and can interact, is ideally constructed for this kind of conversation. It's no surprise, then, that studies conducted in children's homes have found that language interaction during routine caretaking tasks, such as mealtimes, is among the strongest predictors of children's growing language abilities (Hoff-Ginsburg 1991).

The amount and type of conversation at mealtimes varies quite a bit across cultures and social classes (Hall, Nagy, and Linn 1984). But all groups have some amount of talk over meals. In the United States, across different social classes, mealtimes usually include some combination of explanatory talk (answering children's questions, explaining things in their world), narrative talk (storytelling that recounts past events or plans future events), and management talk (managing children's behavior during mealtime). Explanatory and narrative conversations, in which people talk back and forth on a single topic for a period of time, provide the most opportunity for extended discourse (Snow and Beals 2006), which promotes more language learning.

The amount of explanatory and narrative talk at mealtime varies quite a bit from one family to the next, with some families doing quite a bit and other families with preschool-age children doing zero explanatory or narrative talk during a typical mealtime (Beals and Snow 1994). A rich language environment at the early education program's meal table can encourage every child's language development. For children who hear little or no explanatory or narrative talk at home, this stimulation in the early education program can make a crucial difference in the child's language development and overall preparation for later schooling, making up for the lack of language interaction at home.

## ✓ PRACTICE TIP

### Creating Great Mealtime Conversations

*Create joint attention and name the experience.* Especially with infants, start by making sure you and the child are paying attention to the same thing, then comment on it, providing words for the child's experience. By connecting words to the child's experience, you teach those words. "Oh, you see the cup. Are you thirsty?"

*Elaborate on their language.* When children say one or two words, you can answer back by adding to those words. This guarantees joint attention, and helps the child figure out the meaning of the words you have added. "Milk? Ah, you want me to pass the pitcher of milk." "Yes, the casserole has green bits in it, and they are bell pepper."

*Ask real questions.* Some teachers are in the habit of asking "testing questions." These are questions the teacher already knows the answer to, such as, "What color is your watermelon?" A real question is one the teacher does not know the answer to. Children will often enjoy talking more when they can talk about something *they* are the expert in. "Chelsea, what foods does your family grow in your garden?" "Hannah, what is your favorite food?"

*Play with letter sounds.* The meal table is a great place to be playful with words in ways that teach letter sounds. Begin by pointing out words that rhyme: "Here is some corn. Let's name words that have the same ending sound as corn. Yes: born, torn." Nonsense words are okay, too. You can connect sounds to the first letter of a food: "Look, broccoli and beans both start with the letter B. Can you hear the B? Buh-broccoli; Buh-beans."

*Direct the conversation.* Do so in a way that each child gets to speak, but everyone stays on the same topic. You can accomplish this by summarizing what a child has said and asking another child to comment. "Juan's favorite food is tortillas with jam, and Jason likes strawberries. What about you, Margo? What's your favorite food?" Sometimes you may need to remind children of the topic: "Wait, Damon, Reiko was talking about our trip to the farm. Can you tell us what we did next, after seeing the chickens?"

## Mealtime Math

Opportunities for math learning are just about everywhere you look at the meal table. Everything you wish to teach about mathematics—numbers, sets, fractions, simple arithmetic—can be taught while enjoying a nutritious lunch or snack.

- Setting the table provides a concrete example of the *one-to-one correspondence* an understanding of numbers is based on. Ask the children how many plates are needed for the table (they can count the chairs). Then ask how many cups, how many forks. There is always one for each setting, so the numbers are the same.

- *Simple arithmetic,* subtraction and addition, can then enter the discussion. "If Hiroshko wasn't here today, then how many plates would we need? How many cups and forks?" "If Hiroshko's mother and father joined us for lunch, then how many plates would we need?"

- The everyday problem of dividing food or snacks evenly provides the earliest understanding of *fractions* for many children. Start with easy problems, like how to divide three pieces of fruit between two children (cutting one piece in half solves the problem). Work up to harder problems, like how to divide two bagels among three children (each child gets one-third of each bagel, which is a concrete example of the lowest common denominator solution). Be sure to describe in words the math the children have done. Savvy teachers sometimes create problems on purpose, just so the children have to work through the solution. You might have enough bagels for all the children, but putting out too few gives them a problem they will literally want to sink their teeth into!

## Science Learning with Food

Most of *science learning* in the early childhood years concerns knowledge of the natural world, and in particular, an understanding of transformations in materials. Food provides the first and most compelling examples of this, as it combines both natural science (where does food come from?) and basic chemistry (how does it change when it is cooked?).

Children are fascinated by learning about the source of our foods. Even though gardens take weeks to grow, many early childhood programs use them as an activity that helps children study the natural world. Because plants change too slowly to really see, children can keep track of changes by measuring plant height each week (and putting it on a chart), or photographing the plant each week (and posting the photos on a chart), or planting new seeds at one week intervals so the week-by-week progress can be directly seen. Using fast-growing plants, like beans and radishes, is a good idea. The classroom science takes on new meaning when children see similar beans in the grocery market or radishes in their salads and, most important, when they harvest and eat their own produce.

The *Early Sprouts* gardening and nutrition curriculum for early childhood programs by Karrie Kalich, Dottie Bauer, and Deirdre McPartlin (2009, 13) takes a "seed-to-table" approach to teaching children the basics of appreciating food. The authors state that planting seeds helps set the stage for children to understand the source of the foods they eat, and "by beginning with seeds and seedlings, *Early Sprouts* provides a connection to the natural world that is missing in many children's lives."

Every form of cooking can be considered a science experiment. Like all good science education, having the children actually do the cooking themselves (to the extent possible) is the best way for them to learn. In addition to measuring and counting, have the children observe how things change when they are mixed or cooked. Many preschoolers will be mystified by something as simple as a piece of bread turning into

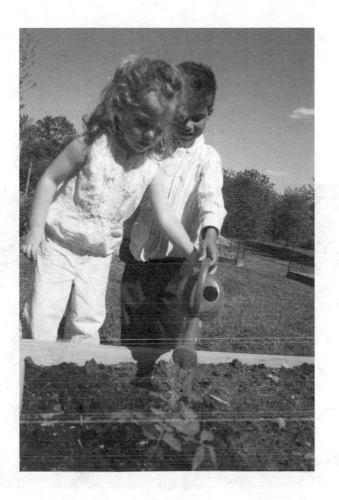

toast. Ask them, "Is it still a piece of bread?" Compare a slice of toasted bread with a slice of bread, and talk about what has happened. The change from bread into toast (or from fruit juice to fruit popsicles or from dough into pretzels, for example) seems uninteresting to adults but can be unexpected, fascinating, and even confusing to young children.

At a young age, children believe that when the appearance of something changes, it has become something different. For example, preschoolers often believe that if a man puts on a dress, he will become a woman; or if a line of raisins is spread out into a longer line, there will be more raisins; or if a sandwich is cut into more pieces, there is more sandwich. Adults know this is illogical, but young children must learn about the *conservation of identity* through their own experiences. Child psychologist Jean Piaget first described conservation of identity (Ginsburg and Opper 1988). His work on children's thinking changed early childhood education practices around the world (DeVries and Kohlberg 1987).

Cooking provides the exact kinds of experiences, and with natural materials, that can help preschoolers learn what changes and what doesn't when materials go through transformations such as being cut, mixed, cooked, or frozen. The simplest of questions can prompt interesting and useful discussions. If we cut it into slices, is this still an apple? If we crush the graham crackers into powder, what does it begin to look like? If we pour all the juice into this tall, thin glass, is there more juice than before?

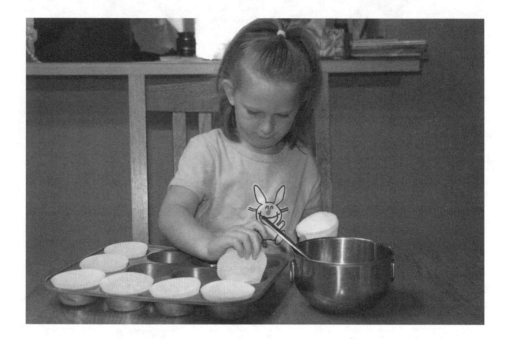

PROMISING PRACTICE

## Following the Cycle of Food from Production to Preparation

### WHAT WE SAW

In one child care program, the children went on a field trip to an apple orchard where they picked apples. The next day, back at the center, the teacher sliced apples into thin sections and the children spread a thin layer of peanut butter or cream cheese on each slice for snacktime. They also made applesauce, with the children helping mash the cooked apples.

## WHAT IT MEANS

At any age, there is no substitute for learning by doing. These children learned where apples come from (trees) before showing up at the table. Seeing the many ways an apple can be changed before being eaten helps children begin to wrestle with *conservation of identity*. Seeing the whole apple and then the slices of apple (or applesauce) is not enough. Children learn best when they see the transformations with their own eyes and make those transformations happen with their own hands.

PROMISING PRACTICE

# Cooking

## WHAT WE SAW

Six children at a time came to the kitchen to help cook. They were standing around a child-sized table in the kitchen, helping to mix and then stir the dry and wet ingredients together to make muffins. Each took a turn, and the cook showed one child how to hold the side of the bowl while stirring, saying "Use your helper hand, like this." The cook also had three smaller bowls, each containing a small amount of muffin batter that was too wet and runny, or too dry and hard, or just the right consistency. She asked the children to compare the batter in the bowls and tell her if each was the right wetness, like the batter in the large bowl. They added a little flour or milk to adjust the batter until it was the same in all three bowls.

## WHAT IT MEANS

This was a large child care program that had a kitchen staff. Over time, the cooks had become part of the instructional staff. Along with the bus driver and the janitor, they attended staff meetings and trainings and were asked how they could incorporate the early childhood curriculum and teaching methods into their work. The cooks had become experts on not only nutrition and cooking but also on early childhood science learning in the kitchen!

## ✓ PRACTICE TIP

### Plant a Friendship Garden

Have you ever made stone soup with children, in which each child follows the *Stone Soup* storybook's theme and contributes an ingredient to create something that everyone can enjoy? How about trying a Friendship Garden? Families bring their favorite vegetable plant for the school or child care program's garden. Every time the families look at the garden, they will see not only the vegetable they enjoy but also the diversity of plants that others enjoy. You could even laminate the child or family's picture and place it on a plant marker by the plant. Taking it one step further, have families write down why they like this vegetable, and create a collage or quilt of pictures of the vegetables with the reasons families like them. It will be a source of conversation and smiles and inspire children to take care of their special family vegetable.

- Provide gardening tools designed for children. Make sure each child has her own tools to use.

- Establish a few simple safety rules.

    - Keep feet on the grass or path, not in the garden.

    - Never pick or eat plants without the teacher telling you that it is safe.

    - Use child tools in a safe way.

- Work with small groups of children (four to eight, depending on their ages).

- Include children as young as eighteen months by having them begin simple garden activities, such as watering plants and digging in soil.

- Start with simple lessons, such as what plants need to live—soil, water, air, and sunshine.

- Let children dig in a pile of soil that contains worms. Investigate how these creatures help the soil.

- Plant gardens in framed wooden beds that are approximately ten feet long, three feet wide, and ten to twelve inches high. Children then have easy access to the gardens without stepping into them.

- Read quality children's books (see further reading at the end of this chapter) to introduce a fruit or vegetable at the time of planting, harvesting, or eating.

- Investigate the six main parts of a plant—roots or tubers, stem, leaves, flower, fruit, and seed—and their roles in helping the plant to grow.

- Grow plants for each of the six main parts of a plant that people eat; for example, carrots, beets, potatoes (roots/tubers); asparagus, celery, rhubarb (stems); spinach, lettuce, kale (leaves); tomatoes, cucumbers, eggplant, strawberries (fruits); broccoli, cauliflower (flowers); sunflowers, peas, corn (seeds).

- Involve children in all phases of gardening, such as planting, mulching, watering, weeding, and harvesting.

- Cook, prepare, and eat the produce outdoors to make it taste extra special.

- Allow children to taste their produce when it's freshly picked and washed, prior to cooking it.

- Plant an herb garden with herbs that can be used for seasoning the produce after it's harvested.

- Create fun and playful gardens, such as a mini gourd tunnel for children to crawl through, a sunflower house for story reading time, and a bean tepee for playing hide-and-seek.

- Develop theme gardens, such as the "salad bowl" or "pizza pie."

- Make a flower garden that will attract butterflies and hummingbirds.

- Brainstorm with children simple recipes for preparing the produce.

- Try preparing a food several different ways: sautéed, boiled, raw, or steamed. Ask children which way they prefer the food prepared and graph their responses.

## Further Reading

### On Research

Larson, Reed W., Angela R. Wiley, and Kathryn R. Branscomb, eds. 2006. *Family mealtime as a context of development and socialization*. New directions for child and adolescent development, no. 111. San Francisco: Jossey-Bass.

Riley, Dave, Mary A. Carns, Joan Klinkner, Ann Ramminger, and Colette Cisco. 2009. *Intellectual development: Connecting science and practice in early childhood settings*. St. Paul, MN: Redleaf Press.

Riley, Dave, Robert R. San Juan, Joan Klinkner, and Ann Ramminger. 2008. *Social and emotional development: Connecting science and practice in early childhood settings*. St. Paul, MN: Redleaf Press.


## On Practice

Branscomb, Kathryn R., and Carla B. Goble. 2008. Infants and toddlers in group care: Feeding practices that foster emotional health. *Young Children* 63 (6): 28–33.

Colker, Laura J. 2005. *The cooking book: Fostering young children's learning and delight*. Washington, DC: National Association for the Education of Young Children.

Dennee, JoAnne, Julia Hand, Jack Peduzzi, and Carolyn Peduzzi. 1996. *In the three sisters garden: Native American stories and seasonal activities for the curious child*. A common roots guidebook. Denver: Food Works.

Jaffe, Roberta, and Gary Appel. 1990. *The growing classroom: Garden-based science*. Parsippany, NJ: Life Lab Science Program.

Kalich, Karrie, Dottie Bauer, and Deirdre McPartlin. 2009. *Early sprouts: Cultivating healthy food choices in young children*. St Paul, MN: Redleaf Press.

Starbuck, Sara, and Maria R. Olthof. 2008. Involving families and community through gardening. *Young Children* 63 (5): 74–79.

Wisconsin Department of Health Services. 2008. Got dirt? Gardening initiative. Nutrition and Physical Activity Program. http://dhs.wisconsin .gov/health/physicalactivity/gotdirt.htm.

This guide to setting up school gardens is available online, or you can order a copy from the Web site.

U.S. Department of Agriculture. Food and Nutrition Service Team Nutrition. 2009. Grow it, try it, like it! Preschool Fun with Fruits and Vegetables. http://teamnutrition.usda.gov.

Preschool fun with fruits and vegetables. This kit has six booklets that feature peaches, strawberries, cantaloupe, spinach, sweet potatoes, and crookneck squash. Order or download from the Team Nutrition Web site.


## Children's Books about Food and Gardening

Anderson, Sara. 2007. *Fruit*. Brooklyn, NY: Handprint Books.

———. 2007. *Vegetables*. Brooklyn, NY: Handprint Books.

Ayres, Katherine. 2007. *Up, down, and around*. Cambridge, MA: Candlewick Press.

Berger, Thomas, and Carla Grillis. 1990. *The mouse and the potato.* Edinburgh: Floris Books.

Bunting, Eve. 1996. *Sunflower house.* San Diego: Harcourt Brace and Co.

———. 1997. *The pumpkin fair.* New York: Clarion Books.

Carle, Eric. 1991. *The tiny seed.* New York: Simon and Schuster.

Cherry, Lynne. 2003. *How the groundhog's garden grew.* New York: Blue Sky Press.

Cole, Henry. 1995. *Jack's garden.* New York: Greenwillow Books.

Doyle, Malachy. 1999. *Jody's beans.* Cambridge, MA: Candlewick Press.

Ehlert, Lois. 1987. *Growing vegetable soup.* San Diego: Harcourt Brace Jovanovich.

———. 1996. *Eating the alphabet.* San Diego: Harcourt Brace.

Fleming, Candace. 2002. *Muncha! Muncha! Muncha!* New York: Atheneum Books.

Florian, Douglas. 1996. *Vegetable garden.* San Diego: Harcourt Brace Jovanovich.

Glaser, Linda. 1992. *Wonderful worms.* Brookfield, CT: Millbrook Press.

Golden Gelman, Rita. 1992. *More spaghetti, I say!* New York: Scholastic.

Grossnickle Hines, Anna. 1986. *Daddy makes the best spaghetti.* New York: Clarion Books.

Hall, Zoe. 1998. *The surprise garden.* New York: Blue Sky Press.

Hoban, Russell. 1964. *Bread and jam for Frances.* New York: Harper and Row.

Jordan, Helene J. 1992. *How a seed grows.* New York: HarperCollins Publishers.

Klinting, Lars. 2006. *Harvey the gardner.* Boston: Kingfisher.

Knight, Joan. 1993. *Bon appetit, Bertie!* London: Houghton Mifflin Company.

Krauss, Ruth. 1945. *The carrot seed.* New York: Harper and Bros.

Pfeffer, Wendy. 2004. *From seed to pumpkin.* New York: HarperCollins.

Prelutsky, Jack. 2007. *In Aunt Giraffe's green garden.* New York: Greenwillow Books/HarperCollins.

Ross, Tony. 1987. *Stone soup.* New York: Dial Books for Young Readers.

Scott, Emily, and Catherine Duffy. 1998. *Dinner from dirt*. Salt Lake City: Gibbs Smith.

Seuss, Dr. 1960. *Green eggs and ham*. New York: Random House.

Sloat, Teri. 2004. *Berry magic*. Anchorage: Alaska Northwest Books.

Vaccaro Seeger, Laura. 2007. *First the egg*. New Milford, CT: Roaring Brook Press.

---

## When Teachers Reflect

### Becoming a Gardener

You have read about how educational and fun gardening can be with children, but what if you have never gardened before and are not sure where to start? Who might give you advice, and who would enjoy helping you?

Perhaps you work in a program with no room to garden outside but are interested in the benefits of growing plants with young children. Your room may not have much natural light or counter space for growing plants. How do you get started? What creative options can you explore? What household recyclable containers could be used to grow plants? How could grandparents, community elders, or others help you with the project? How could you be creative with space to create a classroom growing area?

What worries you about starting to garden with the children? That the plants will grow too slowly? That half the plants will die? Relax. Whatever happens will be a part of nature, and a source for learning.

---

## When Teachers Reflect

### Using Mealtimes More for Learning

Think about the mealtimes in your program. Earlier in this chapter you learned that responsive, well-organized, and well-regulated mealtimes predict better child outcomes in a wide variety of areas. Take time to observe during your mealtimes. Do you see opportunities to teach social skills such as sharing, impulse control, and self-responsibility? Do you think of mealtime as a part of your literacy curriculum? How can you be more intentional about children's learning during this time in a variety of developmental areas? What is one thing you can do differently at mealtime tomorrow?

## When Teachers Reflect

### Partnering with Parents

Teachers of infants and toddlers often have values, beliefs, and training in specific ways to approach feeding and mealtime with children. Here are two examples.

1. Because teachers are competent and like to feel efficient, doing things themselves (setting the table, serving the food, or spoon-feeding a toddler) is often easier and faster than letting children do the same things. Yet we know that emotional health and social skills can be fostered by allowing children to do more for themselves. Consider that in infant and toddler care, up to 80 percent of a teacher's time may be spent dealing with daily routines such as feeding, napping, and toileting.

2. Another consideration is the need for solid communication between parents and caregivers about family customs or beliefs about nutrition and feeding. Sometimes our program policies or values clash with a parent's requests or desires and can become emotionally charged.

Think about a time when you did not agree with a parent on a feeding issue. How did you handle it? What were the beliefs or values underlying your position? How were they different from the parent position? How was the child helped or hurt by the varying viewpoints between teacher and parent? How could the situation be handled more effectively in the future?

# Letter to Families: Dealing with Picky Eaters

**Dear Parent:**

If your child seems overly choosy about what she is willing to eat, ask yourself the following questions:

1. Is my child saying no to foods as a way to establish her independence? This type of behavior is normal for young children as they learn to make more and more decisions for themselves.

2. Is my child's appetite more erratic than it was when she was younger? The rate of growth of a preschooler is not as rapid as it was in infancy and toddlerhood, so it is common for parents to wonder if their child is getting enough food.

In most cases, the best way to deal with a child who seems overly fussy about what she is willing to eat is to relax. Offering a favored food such as dessert for eating vegetables or meat may seem a logical way to encourage a child to eat healthy food. However, research shows it may make the child's eating worse in the long run. Instead, follow these suggestions from a "Nibbles for Health" fact sheet from the U.S. Department of Agriculture (www.fns.usda.gov/tn/Resources/Nibbles/Nibbles_Newsletter_13.pdf).

1. Treat food jags casually, since food jags do not last long anyway.

2. Consider what a child eats over several days, not just at each meal. Most kids eat more of a variety of foods than a parent thinks.

3. Trust your child's appetite rather than force a child to eat everything on the plate. Forcing a child to eat more encourages overeating.

4. Set reasonable time limits for the start and end of a meal, then remove the plate quietly. What is reasonable depends on each child.

From *Rethinking Nutrition* by Susan Nitzke, Dave Riley, Ann Ramminger, and Georgine Jacobs, with Ellen Sullivan, © 2010.

Redleaf Press grants permission to photocopy this page for classroom use.

5. Stay positive and avoid criticizing or calling any child a "picky eater." Children believe what you say!

6. Serve food plain, and respect the "no foods touching" rule if that's important to your child. This will pass.

7. Avoid being a short-order cook by offering the same food for the whole family. Plan at least one food everyone will eat.

8. If a child does not like a certain food, substitute a similar one; instead of squash, offer sweet potatoes.

9. Provide just two or three choices, not a huge array of food. Then let your child decide.

10. Focus on your child's positive eating behavior, not on the food.

From *Rethinking Nutrition* by Susan Nitzke, Dave Riley, Ann Ramminger, and Georgine Jacobs, with Ellen Sullivan, © 2010.

Redleaf Press grants permission to photocopy this page for classroom use.

# 5

# Why We Implement Food and Nutrition Policies

## Observation: Making Jacob's Birthday Special

*"Can I bring cupcakes to school for my birthday?" Jacob, who was soon to be four years old, asked his mom. "Tommy brought a treat for his birthday!" Shawna, Jacob's mom, remembered from family orientation that there was a policy at child care about birthday treats and asked Jacob's teacher for options. Jacob's teacher reminded Shawna the program provided a suggested list of low-sugar birthday treats and snacks in the family handbook. Jacob's teacher also let Shawna know that two children in the class had wheat allergies. Shawna wondered if Jacob's birthday would feel "special" enough, whereupon the teacher explained her classroom's birthday ritual. Everyone sings the school's special birthday song before the morning snack and Jacob gets to pick the book for story time that day. Shawna used the school's fruit snack list to offer Jacob two choices she knew he really liked, and he picked one of his favorites—a fruit and yogurt parfait.*

### Societal Trends and Program Policies

Whether the subject is birthday treats or parking lot etiquette, policies are indispensable in early childhood programs. When they are thoughtfully developed and shared with families and other key stakeholders, policies provide concrete examples of the program's values while minimizing misunderstandings and conflicts that might otherwise disrupt the program's work and the children's learning environment. Parents may wonder why there are so many policies in early childhood settings. Considering that many children spend eight hours or more per day in a setting away from home and eat two meals and two snacks, it is imperative that nutrition be taken seriously. In the past, nutrition care may have been provided more by parents, grandparents, and extended relatives. Now nutrition care rests also with early childhood professionals.

The care and nurturing of one generation toward another is a societal issue that varies across the United States and throughout the world. The future of any society depends on the ability and commitment of that society to foster the health and well-being of the next generation (National Scientific Council on the Developing Child 2007). The role of food in the care and nurturing of children has deep roots in family systems and includes the roles and influence of extended family.

As the role of women in society has changed and the participation of women in the workforce has increased, the corresponding need for out-of-home care for children has increased proportionately. In 1960, only 37.7 percent of women were members of the workforce. Compare that to 2007, when 59.3 percent of women were either employed or searching for employment (U.S. Department of Labor 2008). A study by the National Women's Law Center further shows that in 2006 64 percent of women with children under age six and 56 percent of women with infants (under age one) were in the labor force (2008). As a result, the historical traditions and responsibilities of family meals are shared between the child's home and his or her early childhood program. Therefore, there is a need to look at partnerships between families and child care professionals to ensure the nutrition needs of children are met.

Nutritional health is a core building block of young children's quality care and nurturing. Eating—along with warmth, shelter, and sleep—is a basic biological need, and healthy eating habits are essential to a child's developmental progress. Abraham Maslow (1970), a theorist and leader in the humanistic psychology movement, proposed that only when needs are met can human beings fully develop to their potential (Gonzalez-Mena 2008). Since young children rely on adults to provide healthy meals and snacks, staff in early childhood programs have an ethical responsibility to understand the biological role nutritional health plays in the foundation for further growth and learning in all areas of development.

## Rationale for Developing Nutrition Policies

Early childhood programs must develop appropriate nutrition policies to assist staff in meeting children's health and nutrition needs. Policies act as a guide for orienting and training staff with the information, skills, and attitudes necessary to meet a variety of children's needs. Responsible programs develop policies that directly reflect the specific needs of the families who have children enrolled in their program and that meet their state's regulations. Of course, policies alone will not be effective unless they are thoroughly and consistently shared with families and implemented by staff. Best practice calls for frequent review of policies to evaluate their relevance, effectiveness, and practical implementation. Well-written policies also help staff members deal with a variety of situations in a consistent manner. National early childhood organizations developed nutritional guidelines because they understand how integral they are to quality services for children and families. In turn, these national guidelines are helpful in providing a framework for local nutrition policies.

## Nutritional Guidance from National Early Childhood Organizations

Two of the most well-known national early childhood organizations to include solid nutritional guidelines are the National Association for the Education of Young Children (NAEYC) and the U.S Department of Health and Human Services. Portions of those guidelines for family-centered practice, nutritional programming, and food safety are listed in the table of NAEYC Accreditation Criteria (2007) and Head Start Performance Standards (U.S Department of Health and Human Services 2006) that follows.

| | NAEYC Accreditation Criteria | Head Start Performance Standards |
|---|---|---|
| Family-Centered Practices | Written menus are posted for families<br><br>Procedures are in place to support breastfeeding<br><br>Families are provided with documentation of food consumed by infants and children with disabilities | Staff and families work together to identify each child's nutritional needs<br><br>Families and relevant community agencies are involved in planning, implementing, and evaluating nutritional services<br><br>Parent nutrition education opportunities are provided |

|  | NAEYC Accreditation Criteria | Head Start Performance Standards |
|---|---|---|
| Nutritional Programming | Teaching staff sit and eat with children and engage in conversation<br><br>Snacks are served family style when possible<br><br>Teaching staff engage in reflective practice to improve their practices | Food is not used as punishment or reward, and each child is encouraged, but not forced, to eat or taste the food<br><br>Adults eat family style, with all toddlers and preschool children sharing the same menu to the extent possible<br><br>A variety of foods are served, which broadens each child's food experiences |
| Food Safety | Children under four years are not given foods that may cause choking, such as popcorn, whole grapes, and hard pretzels<br><br>Formula or human milk is warmed in 120 degree water for 5 minutes or less<br><br>Food is prepared in accordance with the USDA CACFP guidelines | Children under one year old should not be fed honey<br><br>In programs that serve infants and toddlers there must be proper storage and handling of breast milk and formula<br><br>Evidence of compliance is posted, along with all applicable federal, state, tribal, and local food safety and sanitation laws |

Appendix 3 shows an example of rotating Head Start menus that can be adapted for various early childhood programs.

## State Early Learning Standards

State early learning standards provide a framework for early education professionals to expand their understanding of the importance of child development and developmentally appropriate practices in collaboration across all settings, including child care, Head Start, public schools, health departments, libraries, family resource centers, and home visitation programs. These standards can help families understand the general developmental continuum of eating and feeding behaviors as well as implement strategies to help their children with them. Staff from various programs and settings might find the standards useful to discuss the consistency of adult interactions during meals and snacks. You can review your state's early learning standards at http://nccic.acf.hhs.gov/pubs/goodstart/elgwebsites.html. See appendix 1 for further explanations and examples of early learning standards.

## Ethical Considerations

Parents, early education professionals, communities, and policy makers have an ethical obligation to use the growing body of evidence on brain research as well as child development to craft and deliver policies that not only protect children from harm but also promote optimum physical, cognitive, social, and emotional growth. The importance of nutrition to these areas of growth is already recognized in several federal programs, such as the Child and Adult Care Food Program (CACFP); the Special Supplemental Nutrition Program for Women, Infants, and Children (WIC); and Extension's Expanded Food and Nutrition Education Program (EFNEP) (Aronson 2002). Proper nutrition is important to brain development and, along with nurturing interactions and rich experiences, promotes developmental growth. An understanding of key nutrients in children's diets is as important as teaching colors, numbers, or social skills.

Early education programs are in a unique position to partner with families in a community approach to influence the overall health of children. Parents do not always know what is nutritionally sound for their young children, and they rely on early childhood professionals and nutritionists to guide them through the early years of parenting. NAEYC has developed an Ethical Code of Conduct as a professional guide to ethical practices for early learning professionals (Feeney and Freeman 1999). Ethical dilemmas always exist, and issues around food are no exception. The NAEYC Ethical Code of Conduct outlines ideals and principles regarding ethical responsibilities to children, families, colleagues, community, and society. The code of conduct can be helpful as a resource to guide policy development, a framework for difficult decisions, and a tool for staff training. Nutritionists and early childhood staff may find the code useful in evaluating nutritional practices for children with special eating needs and discussing options with families.

## Cultural and Individual Differences

People naturally form beliefs and attitudes about child rearing based partly on how they were raised and how those around them reinforced these practices. Professionals can broaden their perspectives by using a wider lens to view the possibilities of child rearing around the world. This approach of looking at families as a continuously running movie, rather than a snapshot in time, helps to develop different viewpoints.

In order to provide the most successful experiences for children, early childhood staff and parents must work together. It will usually require more effort by staff to consider the family perspective in child rearing, communicate respectfully when there are differences, and settle on a resolution that is best for the child. Consider the differences between the individualist and collectivist approaches to child rearing described in the table that follows (Gonzalez-Mena 2008). While these are generalizations, they highlight conflicts in the early education practices of caring for and educating young children that may be encountered between families from collectivist cultures and professionals from individualist cultures (typically most Western cultures, including the United States).

| Individualist Values for Children | Collectivist Values for Children |
|---|---|
| Independence: Children are encouraged to feed themselves, even though their faces, hands, and clothing may get messy | Interdependence between adults and children: Adults assist in feeding children to conserve food, prevent mess, save time, or nurture relationships |
| Self-help skills: Children are encouraged to pour their own milk | Receiving help with tasks: The milk is poured so it is not spilled and wasted |
| Individualized praise for accomplishment of tasks: Adult claps and cheers when child finally tries broccoli after many attempts | Modesty and humbleness with personal accomplishment: Children are expected to eat the food that is provided for them |

Other cultural differences may be evident, such as when families follow a vegetarian or vegan diet, have dietary needs based on their culture, or object to children playing with food in the dramatic play or art area. These differences will not be viewed as unreasonable opinions or requests if programs consider the perspective of the family:

- Has food been scarce in their family or country of origin?
- Are certain foods avoided because of a medical condition?
- Are there allergies or food intolerances?
- Do religious or personal beliefs contribute to their requests?

It is helpful to think about these questions when developing policies for your program. Does your enrollment form ask questions about eating routines and habits? While a program must have some consistent guidelines, are these based on the predominant culture or experiences of those who wrote the policies or direct the program? Since meals and snacks are a regular part of every day, it is worth taking a closer look at how program policies are written and whether they truly represent the diversity of staff and families. New staff orientation and regular, continuing education on implementing policies with sensitivity are important components of honoring individual and cultural differences.

## ✓ PRACTICE TIP

### The Rule of Six

Judy Brown (2007) proposes a reflective practice tip called the Rule of Six, which she learned from Paula Underwood (1994), a Native American wise woman. This tip encourages careful listening to each perspective and deeper understanding of the reasons behind how each person might feel or how their experiences brought them to a certain point of view. To use the Rule of Six, take an issue of concern or disagreement and then think of six different ways to interpret or explain it. It helps to think of the perspective as coming from the viewpoint of a

- child
- parent or guardian
- teacher
- administrator
- non-English speaker
- community member

Discuss the perspectives of each stakeholder to gain better understanding of the situation. This process could be worked through at a staff meeting to help everyone develop the ability to look at something with different perspectives. All views should be honored and respected as potentially valid. Weigh perspectives with program policies and regulatory standards to create and implement quality practices that honor diversity.

PROMISING PRACTICE

## Grumpy Sammy

### WHAT WE SAW

The teachers in a three-year-old classroom asked their director for help with Sammy, a child in their program who had started exhibiting disruptive behaviors every morning. The director agreed to observe in the classroom to gather more information. The director watched the grandmother drop off Sammy with a loving good-bye. Sammy adjusted to the classroom but with the passing minutes he began to take toys from other children and push children out of his way when he wanted to get to an activity. At snacktime, the director noticed Sammy eating great quantities of food, after which his behavior was noticeably improved.

The director then asked the teachers if they had talked with the parents lately. The teachers recalled that Sammy's parents were going through a divorce and Sammy was staying with his grandmother for a while. The director then asked if the grandmother knew about the nutrition policies of the center. The teachers assumed the parents would have communicated that information. The director recommended that the teachers call the parents to let the grandparent know snack was not served until 9:00 AM and Sammy might need more to eat before he came to the center. Once the parents and grandmother knew about this policy, Sammy received more food before he came to the program and his behavior improved.

### WHAT IT MEANS

Sammy's basic nutritional needs were not being met, and as a result, his behavior was changing. Think about how it feels to be very hungry. Do you think as well when you are hungry as when you are not? Might you say or do things not typical of you when you are hungry? Adults can take action when hungry, but young children rely on adults to recognize and attend to their needs. Do not assume that because parents have been given program policies they will remember and communicate them to other caregivers. This family was going through a stressful time, and Sammy's behavior could have been attributed to that situation. With further observation and questioning, however, it was discovered that the meeting of a basic need helped Sammy be more successful in the classroom.

## Policies on Food Allergies and Intolerances

As mentioned in chapter 2, early childhood settings are in a unique position to partner with families in identifying and responding to food allergies and intolerances. Some children may eat two out of three meals per day, five days per week, in an early childhood setting. Staying in close contact with families about health issues benefits the child. In addition, most state licensing departments require a child health exam along with a health history that must be updated at regular intervals.

It is critical that program policies include the following processes and procedures:

- All staff must know allergies of all children.

- Allergies must be posted in a conspicuous but confidential manner.

- Instructions from the parent and physician must at all times be kept with the teacher supervising the child.

- Emergency equipment, such as epinephrine injection devices (EpiPens), must be both readily available and secured from children's reach.

- Staff must be trained in emergency procedures for responding to allergies.

- If a child is severely allergic to a particular food, it should not be served anywhere in the entire setting.

- Parents should be sent regular reminders to let staff members know about allergies.

**PROMISING PRACTICE**

## Peanut-Free

### WHAT WE SAW

A family child care provider had a two-year-old child who was severely allergic to peanuts. Because his policies indicated he would provide meals for all children, the parents agreed to help him adapt his menus not only to keep their child safe but also to educate the other children and parents as well. The parents belonged to a local support group for parents of children with food allergies. This support group had gathered a long list of foods that should be avoided because they contained peanuts or were in facilities that also prepared peanut products. Although the list was helpful, it wasn't clear about how to adapt menus from it. The parents called a nutrition consultant at the state Department of Education to ask for help. As a result, a complete set of menus were developed that met USDA CACFP guidelines. Any child care provider could use the menus along with some educational activities for young children in their program to help the children understand how some foods are good for us and some foods make some of us sick. The menus were distributed to other families of the family child care and also distributed in a statewide early education newsletter.

### WHAT IT MEANS

This provider saw his role in partnership with the parents, and by remaining open to change, he helped other children, families, and providers. This situation was viewed as both a learning and teaching opportunity that brought in grassroots and expert involvement. The parents could feel more confident that their child was safe, the provider did not have to worry as much about possible life-threatening reactions for the child, and a systematic approach was taken to increase family child care professionals' knowledge about creative solutions to food allergies.

## Writing Health and Nutrition Policies

When writing or revising health and nutrition policies for an early childhood program, there are key items to research and remember before starting:

1. Know your state licensing regulations regarding food and nutrition as they apply to your program.

2. Gather family information, such as traditions and special needs, either through direct discussions with parents or through a family nutrition survey.

3. Assemble an inclusive team of families, caregivers representing all age groups of children, nutritionists, food

preparation staff, administrators, and other experts, such as pediatricians, to assure cross-sector representation.

4. Keep the policies general enough to incorporate groups of children, while making provisions for the specific needs of individual children.

5. Note the general areas to be covered, including planning and practices of nutrition services, production and serving of meals and snacks, family needs, food safety, and sanitation.

## Policies on Meal Content and Menus

Policies should include the recommended amounts of foods from each food group for both meals and snacks. A meal should include milk or another good source of calcium like yogurt; meat, beans, or similar foods with protein; fruits and vegetables; and a grain food (for example, bread, cereal, rice, or pasta). A snack should include two different food groups. See appendix 2 for more information on meal and snack choices for early childhood programs, as established by the USDA for CACFP.

Whether the program provides breakfast and lunch or it is the responsibility of families to provide them, program policies should require that the meals contain all the nutrients needed for growing children. Be sure to also include adequate training and a list of resources and references staff may consult in meeting their responsibilities as stated in the policies.

## Meeting Special Feeding and Dietary Needs

Procedures for identifying special eating requirements and providing for children with them need to be addressed. Policies should include a meeting with the primary staff person and the children's family to determine the best way to meet the child's special dietary and eating needs. The policy should also include when and how this is to be accomplished.

## Special Policies for Infants and Toddlers

Chapters 1 through 3 discuss recommendations for infant feeding, the introduction of solid food, and adaptations for special needs. It is imperative that families of infants and toddlers are in agreement with your feeding policies and practices. Always include in the policies ways to encourage using breast milk, and provide time and a place for breast pumping and breast-feeding.

## Food Policy Recommendations

Here are additional recommendations to consider when developing health and nutrition policies:

- Eliminate products with little or no nutritional value (for example, soda pop, fruit flavored drinks, gelatin desserts) and items that pose choking risks (for example, chewing gum, whole grapes).

- Address how and where food is to be purchased and stored. Make sure the food is purchased from reputable sources and only includes products that have not expired. Also, ensure that products are sealed and there is no damage to their containers before the purchase. Food needs to be stored according to the products' directions, as well as USDA guidelines.

- Establish detailed procedures to maintain a sanitary and clean food environment. This includes hand washing and sanitizing the utensils, dishes, cooking area, eating spaces, and so on (see appendix 4).

- Take precautions for children and staff safety.

- Provide procedures on how meals, snacks, and beverages will be served (family style, family provided, or teacher served, as discussed in chapter 3).

- Determine eating arrangements for meals and snacks. Clearly explain the roles of the teachers and the children. Recommend utensils that should be used to serve and eat different foods. Describe what is expected from the teacher, including manners, conversation, food serving, and sharing food. Explain acceptable ways for setting the table and involving children in meal or snack preparations.

- Set procedures for cleaning up after meals, snacks, and beverages. Sanitation is very important throughout preparation, eating, and cleanup. Implement precise policies regarding handling trash, composting, storing leftover food, and sanitizing surfaces.

- Explain expectations for personal hygiene, including what is expected of staff and children for hand washing, washing faces, and brushing teeth after meals.

- Decide how to handle desserts and treats. Families and teachers may have varying opinions on giving sugary treats to children. Policies should address birthdays, holiday parties, and other events for which treats are sometimes brought from home. Regulating sugary treats can be a challenge for programs; however, it is necessary to minimize foods and beverages with sugar. If treats are allowed, the sizes of treat portions should be small and they should be a rarity rather than a daily, or even weekly, occurrence.

- Make provisions for large-motor activities. Exercise is an important part of a nutrition policy. The movement plans should include both outdoor and indoor options. (See chapter 2 and appendix 8).

- Clarify staff expectations regarding the importance of acting as good role models for children. For example, even though a staff member may not like milk and may prefer soda instead, she should not be drinking soda in front of the children.

**MISTAKEN PRACTICE**

## Using a Sweet Treat as a Reward for Eating Other, More Nutritious Foods

### WHAT WE SAW

A two-year-old child brought homemade cupcakes for a treat in the classroom one day. The teachers instructed the toddlers they needed to eat all of the three crackers and cup of fruit in front of them before they would get a cupcake.

### WHAT IT MEANS

Giving a sweet treat to children who eat their nutritious food may encourage them to eat the more nutritious food item in the short term, but in the long run, the results are not likely to promote good eating. Research shows that making food A into a reward for eating food B increases the children's preferences for food A, even when A and B are equally liked at the beginning of the experiment (Birch and Fisher 1998; Birch, Marlin, and Rotter 1984).

**WHAT WOULD WORK BETTER**

When possible, the early childhood program should have a policy that promotes nutritious foods or nonfood trinkets as special treats. If that is not possible and a sweet treat is to be served at snacktime, serve the nutritious snack as usual, keeping the sweet treat unmentioned and out of sight. After all the children have been served and had several minutes to eat their snack, bring out the treat and serve it in small portions without enforcing the notion that it is better tasting than the nutritious snack.

## How to Put Policies into Practice

Once a comprehensive food and nutrition policy has been established, the task becomes putting the policy into practice. As mentioned earlier, input from staff who work directly with every age group should be in the written policies. This is the first step in effectively implementing a policy. It is only natural that employees will embrace the policies more fully when they are a part of the decision-making process. Including families will also ensure greater diversity of perspectives and may reduce areas of ambiguity or conflict.

Be sure to review and revise your policies annually in order to keep them current with the needs of enrolled children and families and to accommodate any changes in local regulations. Also, be sure to distribute copies of your policies to all staff members and families. It is not wise to rely on staff to read a policy and then expect them to implement it properly. Changes in policies should be discussed with existing staff and placed into the new-employee orientation handbook.

### Staff Orientation and Training

As one step in successfully implementing your program's policies, several in-service trainings should be held during the work day. Trainers should include experts in the field as well as the program director. Set up workshops with presenters who are not promoting specific products or brands. For example, invite a pediatric dietitian from a hospital or your state licensing representative. Make sure each presenter has had time to review your policies, provide input, and discuss with the director the rationale for the policies in place.

Before the training begins, serve a few samples of tasty snacks or side dishes that meet the program's food and nutrition policies. Everyone loves food. Serving doughnuts sends a contradictory message and can negate the staff's understanding that your program is committed to good nutritional standards.

Trainings for staff should be interactive and encourage the staff's creativity. Activities might include cooking various recipes, distributing a section of the policies to small groups and asking them to brainstorm ways to overcome any obstacles to that practice, or asking staff to demonstrate ways to complete tasks or procedures in the policies. Programs might videotape the director completing a food task. During the training, the staff may watch the video for any intentional or unintentional errors. With a little planning and effort, trainings can be fun and creative.

In-services on policies need to be presented to each new employee. Neglecting to train all staff can result in employees ignoring sections of policies because they have forgotten them, find them inconvenient, or assume they are outdated, unimportant, or irrelevant. Repeat nutrition in-services as new staff members are hired or at least every two years in order to update nutrition information and keep policies foremost in the caregivers' minds.

## Involving Families and Community

Educating families and children about the food and nutrition policies is helpful to get everyone on board. One way to do this is to have a nutrition tasting party with families in the evening. Samples of acceptable treats from home may be available for tasting and recipes distributed to families. Families and staff can learn that special events do not necessarily require sweets to be fun. Family education may also include the guest speakers mentioned above for staff trainings, with a focus on the family's role and concerns about child nutrition.

Involving the community in your healthy food and nutrition program can be fun and help staff and children continue to learn more about nutrition. Teachers or students from a local community college's culinary department, restaurant chefs, and your local WIC program representative are often pleased to set up a cooking experience in a classroom for children. The produce manager from a nearby grocery store may be an enjoyable and informative guest for a classroom of three- to five-year-olds. Ask parents to come into the classroom and cook their favorite nutritious dish with the children. Such guests may offer great opportunities for both teachers and children to learn more about healthy foods, including where they originate and how to best prepare them.

Physical activity goes hand-in-hand with good food and nutrition for promoting children's health in your program's policy statements. Be sure families and staff understand the importance of daily activities that build skills and involve physical movement.

## Further Reading

### On Research

Birch, Leann, and William Dietz, eds. 2008. *Eating behaviors of the young child: Prenatal and postnatal influences on healthy eating.* Elk Grove Village, IL: American Academy of Pediatrics.

Lucarelli, Patti. 2002. Raising the bar for health and safety in child care. *Pediatric Nursing* 22 (3): 239–41, 291.

Marcon, Rebecca A. 2003. Research in review. Growing children: The physical side of development. *Young Children* 58 (1): 80–87.

### On Practice

American Dietetic Association, Society for Nutrition Education, and American School Food Service Association. 2004. Joint position on nutrition services: An essential component of comprehensive school health programs. www.eatright.org/ada/files/Servicesnp.pdf.

Fletcher, Janice, Laurel Branen, and Elizabeth Price. 2005. Building mealtime environments and relationships: An inventory for feeding young children in group settings. University of Idaho School of Family and Consumer Sciences. www.ag.uidaho.edu/feeding/pdfs/BMER.pdf.

This booklet includes twelve topic areas arranged in three clusters. Users may rate any or all of the twelve topic areas for a comprehensive review of mealtime practices in a center or room.

Nutrition in childcare: The best of healthy childcare. *Healthy Childcare.* www.healthychild.net/nutritionpub.html.

Available from Healthy Child Publications, this set of newsletter articles by various experts is a comprehensive nutrition resource for child care and early education programs.

Sanders, Stephen. 2002. *Active for life: Developmentally appropriate movement programs for young children.* Washington, DC: National Association for the Education of Young Children.

U.S. Department of Agriculture Food and Nutrition Service Team Nutrition. 2002. Making Nutrition Count for Children—Nutrition Guidance for Child Care Homes. http://teamnutrition.usda.gov/library.html.

This booklet from the USDA's Team Nutrition explains children's growth and development and how they are related to children's nutrient needs. The information is designed to convey key concepts from MyPyramid, the Dietary Guidelines for Americans.

U.S. Department of Agriculture Food and Nutrition Service Team Nutrition. 2009. Recipes for child care. http://teamnutrition.usda.gov.

This resource was updated in 2009. It is available from the Team Nutrition Web site.

U.S. Department of Agriculture and U.S. Department of Health and Human Services. 2005. *Nutrition and your health: Dietary guidelines for Americans.* 6th ed. Washington, DC: Department of Health and Human Services. (Note: the 7th edition is expected in 2010.)

U.S. Department of Health and Human Services Administration for Children and Families. Child Nutrition Program Performance Standards for Early Head Start. http://eclkc.ohs.acf.hhs.gov/hslc/resources/ECLKC_Bookstore/PDFs/393A3E2041ECA233EBEE89F8099DDD37.pdf, pages 235–36.

Vagovic, Julia C. 2008. Transformers: Movement experiences for early childhood classrooms. *Young Children* 63:26–32.

Wisconsin Department of Public Instruction. 2008. Wisconsin model early learning standards. Bulletin No. 08065.

---

## When Teachers Reflect

### Developing Positive Attitudes toward Food and Eating

*Your Personal Experiences and Beliefs Regarding Food*

Early childhood educators are in a unique position to work in partnership with families on developing healthy nutrition and lifestyle habits for young children. Mealtimes and snacktimes are relationship-based and require thoughtful and strategic approaches. Food is a basic need of all humans, and the social nature of eating is a key component to the healthy social and emotional development of all children.

Think back to when you were a child. Do you remember mealtimes as a pleasant social experience or a stressful one? Were you forced to eat all of the food on your plate? How did that feel? Did your caregivers model good eating habits for you? Was food used as a punishment or reward?

### Modeling Positive Nutritional Messages

Children learn by observing the adults in their life. Early child-hood staff have ethical responsibilities to children, parents, col-leagues, and society to be professional in their practices. Do you model positive attitudes about food and eating? Even if you do not like a food, do you convey a positive image of the impor-tance of trying new foods? Do you model polite behaviors at mealtime, such as saying thank you and please? Is pleasant con-versation an integral part of meals and snacks? Do you refrain from drinking sodas and eating sweets at work?

### Training in Nutrition-Related Areas

You may feel that nutrition policies only apply to the cooks in your program and that you are too busy to pay attention to them; however, nutrition is interwoven with all areas of healthy development. Consider the following questions related to safety issues. Do your policies include how to handle food to avoid food-borne illness and to accommodate children's allergies and intolerances? How did you work with the family to ensure their child was not exposed to the food allergen? Have you encoun-tered a child with a food allergy? Have you had training in the use of an epinephrine injection device (EpiPen)? What training would you like to receive on food allergies or intolerances?

### Ethical Issues and the Rule of Six

Ethical considerations with food and feeding practices can be an emotional issue between providers and families. Consider the following questions with others in your early childhood pro-gram using the Rule of Six discussed earlier in this chapter:

- Have you encountered an emotionally charged issue involving food? If so, how did you handle it? What might you have done differently?

- How would you handle a parent who complains that putting dried beans in the sensory table is wasteful and says food should only be used for eating?

# Letter to Families

### Did You Know?

Early learning programs are required to provide nutritionally balanced meals and snacks according to federal, state, and local guidelines. These guidelines are designed to help your child receive optimum nutrition to help growth and development.

### Did You Know?

Children develop allergies most commonly in the early childhood years. Allergies can be detected early and controlled. Be sure to let your teacher know if your child has any allergies.

### Did You Know?

Many foods that are associated with treats for birthdays and special holidays contain a high amount of sugar, fat, and calories. Fun and healthy alternatives can be offered to children to create new healthy traditions.

### Nutrition Is an Important Part of Your Child's Development

Early childhood programs look at the "whole child" when planning programs and services. We often think about developing the social, cognitive, language, and motor skills of children; however, physical health and development is a foundation for any kind of learning. Join us in providing the best possible nutrition for your child. We post our menus for parents to view and welcome suggestions on healthy foods to serve. We also encourage healthy treats for birthdays and special occasions and want to work with you to keep all of the children healthy and happy.

From *Rethinking Nutrition* by Susan Nitzke, Dave Riley, Ann Ramminger, and Georgine Jacobs, with Ellen Sullivan, © 2010.

Redleaf Press grants permission to photocopy this page for classroom use.

# State Early Learning Standards and Nutrition

## What Are Early Learning Standards?

The National Child Care Information and Technical Assistance Center (2009) describes Early Learning Guidelines (ELG) as "expectations about what children, birth to five years, should know and be able to do during specific age ranges" (http://nccic.acf.hhs.gov/pubs/goodstart/strategicplanning.html). Terminology for ELGs varies across states and may include *early learning standards, learning strands, developmental standards, frameworks, foundations, indicators of progress,* and *benchmarks.* In *Rethinking Nutrition,* the phrase *early learning standards* has been used because it is the common terminology in Wisconsin. Many states use early learning standards to guide the implementation of universal prekindergarten, quality rating systems, or other professional development initiatives. Early learning standards provide a framework for early childhood professionals to be more intentional in how they teach and provide other services for children and families. They are a useful tool to educate families, related professions, and society in general about early learning milestones and quality experiences, adding professional credence to explain *why* you do *what* you do.

## Using Early Learning Standards to Enhance Nutritional Practices

You may wonder how to incorporate the nutritional aspect of early learning standards with other requirements, such as child care licensing, national accreditation, Head Start, Quality Rating Improvement Systems (QRIS), and the Child and Adult Care Food Program (CACFP).

Most quality programs already incorporate the nutritional guidelines from early learning standards through everyday routines, environments, interactions, and activities. We know nutrition is part of looking at the whole child and at how all the areas of development merge and overlap in our professional practices. So the early learning standards concerning nutrition often interrelate with other areas of development. For example, if one of the nutritional early learning standards addresses the foundational skill of a toddler learning to "feed herself with adult assistance" (Wisconsin Model Early Learning Standards Steering Committee 2008, 17), we would set up opportunities for the child to use her fine-motor skills (pincer grasp) to pick up Cheerios by herself and use language skills to talk about how she was using her fingers and her eyes (eye-hand coordination) to find the Cheerios and get them to her mouth. We would also ensure that the child was healthy by washing her hands before and after she ate and that the surface on which she was eating was clean. In addition, we may weave in mathematical concepts, such as the number or size of the Cheerios, and support the child's emotional health by commenting on how she was learning to feed herself. In these ways, nutrition and eating become the vehicle for providing a holistic educational approach.

The tables that follow highlight portions of the nutrition-related performance standards from the state of Wisconsin and learning goals from the state of Florida as aligned with selected guidelines from *Caring for Our Children: National Health and Safety Performance Standards: Guidelines for Out-of-Home Child Care* (American Academy of Pediatrics, American Public Health Association, and National Resources Center for Health and Safety in Child Care 2002). The tables include ideas for interactions, environment, and curricula related to each of the standards as covered in the chapters of this book and are outlined in terms of "what you do" and "why it meets these standards." Explore the early learning standards of the state where you live to see how they align with these examples. Do this at a staff meeting, within a community collaboration setting, or with parents as a strategy to engage them in partnerships and education. To facilitate this process, the National Resource Center for Health and Safety in Child Care and Early Education has developed the comprehensive *Toolkit for Integrating Healthy Physical and Mental Development in Early Learning Guidelines* (2008). The toolkit, including a section on nutrition, is available at http://nrc.uchsc.edu/ELG/elg.htm. Another excellent resource for implementing early learning standards is *Make Early Learning Standards Come Alive: Connecting Your Practice and Curriculum to State Guidelines* by Gaye Gronlund (2006).

To look for a particular state's early learning standards, visit the National Child Care Information Center at http://nccic.acf.hhs.gov/pubs/goodstart/elgwebsites.html, or ask your licensing agency, state Department of Education, or child care resource and referral agency for the information. The full set of *Wisconsin Model Early Learning Standards* can be found at www.collaboratingpartners.com/EarlyLS_docs.htm. The *Florida Birth to Three Learning and Development Standards* (Florida Partnership for School Readiness 2004) can be found at www.floridajobs.org/earlylearning/downloads/pdf/birth_to_3book.pdf. The Florida *Three-, Four-, and Five-Year-Olds Performance Standards* can be found at www.floridajobs.org/earlylearning/oel_performance.html.

## Program Practices That Exemplify Early Learning Standards from Two States: Feeding Infants on Demand

| *Caring for Our Children* Standard 4.013: Feeding Infants on Demand with Feeding by a Consistent Caregiver<br>Caregivers shall feed infants on demand unless the parent and the child's health care provider give written instructions otherwise. Whenever possible, the same caregiver shall feed a specific infant for most of that infant's feedings. | |
|---|---|
| **Wisconsin Model Early Learning Performance Standards A.EL.1d:**<br>Demonstrates behaviors to meet self-help and physical needs. Health encompasses emerging knowledge and practices related to health, safety, and nutrition that promote physical well-being. . . . Good physical health and motor development allow for full participation in learning experiences.<br><br>[The child] physically and verbally indicates a need for food. | **Florida Birth to Three Learning and Developmental Standard H.S./CFR 1304.23(a)(1)-(a)(4): Shows characteristics of nutritional health**<br>Good nutrition is necessary for optimal physical, social, and emotional development. Young infants are dependent on their parents, caregivers, and teachers to ensure that their nutritional needs are met in a consistent, predictable, and appropriate fashion. Good nutritional health is evident when young infants are:<br><br>• breast-feeding, if appropriate. |
| **What You Do** | |
| • Observe cues from infants, noting what verbal and physical behaviors indicate hunger or satiety.<br>• Communicate with parents frequently about feeding amounts, behaviors, and challenges.<br>• Provide a relaxing, private space for families to breast-feed their infants. | |
| **Why It Meets These Standards** | |
| • Understanding the individual temperaments of each child is key to building a trusting relationship that assures the child's needs will be met.<br>• Children rely on the adults in their lives to provide consistent care for them and to adjust strategies as the needs of the children change.<br>• Breast-feeding promotes the physical and emotional health of infants. Supporting families in this practice honors solid nutrition research and promotes parent-child attachment. | |

# Program Practices That Exemplify Early Learning Standards from Two States: Encouraging Self-Feeding by Toddlers

### *Caring for Our Children* Standard 4.024: Encouraging Self-Feeding by Toddlers

Caregivers shall encourage toddlers to hold and drink from a cup, to use a spoon, and to use their fingers for self-feeding.

| Wisconsin Model Early Learning Performance Standards A.EL.1d: | Florida Birth to Three Learning and Developmental Standard H.S./CFR 1304.23(a)(1)(a)(4): Shows characteristics of nutritional health |
|---|---|
| Health encompasses emerging knowledge and practices related to health, safety, and nutrition that promote physical well-being. … Good physical health and motor development allow for full participation in learning experiences.<br><br>[The child] feeds self with adult assistance. | Good nutrition is necessary for optimal physical, social, and emotional development. Young infants are dependent on their parents, caregivers, and teachers to ensure that their nutritional needs are met in a consistent, predictable, and appropriate fashion. Good nutritional health is evident when young infants are:<br><br>• beginning to be introduced to a variety of solid foods. |

## What You Do

- While the children are seated at low tables with sturdy small chairs, sit at their level and model how to eat the same foods the toddlers are trying.
- Offer child-sized utensils to children so they can practice placing food on them while being allowed to use their fingers to eat when necessary.

## Why It Meets These Standards

- Children learn how to chew food and pace their eating by watching adults. When high chairs are replaced with appropriately sized tables and chairs, children can eat with their caregivers as a community and learn positive nutritional habits at a young age.
- It may be a bit messier to allow young children to feed themselves, but it is through this practice that they develop the eye-hand coordination to place food on a utensil and successfully direct it to their mouths. This is a great way to help develop fine-motor skills.

## Program Practices That Exemplify Early Learning Standards from Two States: Portions for Toddlers and Preschoolers

| | |
|---|---|
| *Caring for Our Children* **Standard 4.023: Portions for Toddlers and Preschoolers**<br>The facility shall serve toddlers and preschoolers small-sized portions and shall permit them to have one or more additional servings as needed to meet the needs of the individual child. | **Florida Birth to Three Learning and Developmental Standard H.S./CFR 1304.23(a)(1)-(a)(4): Shows characteristics of nutritional health**<br>The independence and confidence of older toddlers can be seen in their desires to select foods and take charge of their feeding. The supporting and redirecting role of parents, caregivers, and teachers must be exercised with care and patience. Older toddlers show that they are being provided with healthy diets by: |
| **Wisconsin Model Early Learning Performance Standards A.EL.1d:**<br>Health encompasses emerging knowledge and practices related to health, safety, and nutrition that promote physical well-being. . . . Good physical health and motor development allow for full participation in learning experiences.<br><br>[The child] feeds self with proficiency. | • participating, with encouragement, in fixing their own snacks, such as peeling a banana or spreading peanut butter on a cracker. |

### What You Do

- Serve family-style meals and help children take one spoonful and fill their glass halfway.
- Communicate with parents about the child's likes and dislikes, allergies, and food intolerances. Review policies with parents when appropriate. Honor parents' perspectives on food and feeding styles.

### Why It Meets These Standards

- Family-style meals not only teach about impulse control and community sharing, but also help children practice portion control, which can lead to lifelong healthy habits. When children control their own portions, they tend to eat less and more readily try new foods.
- Since mealtimes are an important part of every day, communicating with parents about nutrition helps ensure that the developmental needs of every child are addressed. Being aware of medical and cultural issues regarding food and feeding styles helps provide consistency for the child.

# Program Practices That Exemplify Early Learning Standards from Two States: Socialization during Meals

## *Caring for Our Children* Standard 4.031: Socialization during Meals

Caregivers shall sit at the table and shall eat the meal or snack with the children. Family-style meal service shall be encouraged, except for infants and for very young children who require that an adult feed them. The adult(s) shall encourage social interaction and conversation about the concepts of color, quantity, number, temperature of food, and events of the day. Extra assistance and time shall be provided for slow eaters. Eating should be an enjoyable experience at the facility and at home.

| Wisconsin Model Early Learning Performance Standards A.EL.1d: | Florida Birth to Three Learning and Developmental Standard H.S./CFR 1304.23(a)(1)-(a)(4): Shows characteristics of nutritional health |
|---|---|
| Health encompasses emerging knowledge and practices related to health, safety, and nutrition that promote physical well-being. . . . Good physical health and motor development allow for full participation in learning experiences.<br><br>[The child] uses appropriate table etiquette or manners during mealtimes. | Five-year-olds show awareness of many health issues, especially when these relate to their own experiences. Although they still need reminders to follow good health practices, they are beginning to understand the rationale for these practices. Children show their awareness of these issues by:<br><br>• naming healthy snacks/foods. |

## What You Do

- During mealtimes, talk about where food comes from and its textures, tastes, smells, colors, shapes, and health benefits.
- Model good table manners for children, such as saying "thank you" and "please." When children talk with their mouths full of food, calmly say, "Chew first, then talk." Talk about how you are wiping your mouth with a napkin or pushing in your chair when you leave the table.

## Why It Meets These Standards

- Mealtimes are rich educational opportunities. Weave in mathematical, scientific, linguistic, social, motor, and practical concepts and skills. Mealtime is an opportunity for learning that happens several times a day.
- Early childhood professionals work with children from a variety of backgrounds, cultures, and lifestyles. The ability to model polite behavior not only benefits the children but also may extend into families and community ties.

# Federal Nutrition Regulations and Programs

This appendix explores various programs and federal requirements. You may want to contact the appropriate agency in your state, since regulations stricter than those required by the Federal Food and Nutrition Services may apply, and states contract with individual institutions to provide payment when requirements are met. For further information concerning each of these programs administered in your state, visit the USDA Food and Nutrition Service Web page on child nutrition programs at www.fns.usda.gov/cnd/Contacts/StateDirectory.htm.

## Special Milk Program for Child Care Institutions

The purpose of the Special Milk Program is to encourage the consumption of milk by children in child care, summer camps, homeless feeding sites, and outside-of-school-hours care centers. Participating institutions receive federal reimbursement for each half-pint of milk served to children through eighteen years of age. Public and nonprofit child care institutions, outside-of-school-hours care centers, and other agencies that provide services to children and are not participating in the Child and Adult Care Food Program (CACFP) are eligible to participate in the Special Milk Program. A nonprofit institution must maintain an IRS tax-exempt status 501(c) (3).

USDA regulations require substitutions or modifications in the Special Milk Program for children who are considered to have a disability that restricts their diets. To comply with the Rehabilitation Act of 1973, the Americans with Disabilities Act (ADA) and the USDA nondiscrimination regulation 7 CFR 15b, a child with a disability must be provided substitutions when the child's need for substitutions is supported by a statement signed by a licensed physician. An institution may receive reimbursement for the substituted beverages listed on a physician's statement for a child with special dietary needs.

For further information, contact the agency responsible for the administration of the Special Milk Program in your state or the office of the USDA Food and Nutrition Service Public Information Staff at 703-305-2286 or 3101 Park Center Drive, Room 914, Alexandria, VA 22302. State agency contact information can be found at www.fns.usda .gov/cnd/Contacts/StateDirectory.htm.

## CACFP

The CACFP is one of the USDA Food and Nutrition Service programs that provides financial assistance for nutritious meals and snacks served to children in child care centers, family day care homes, emergency homeless shelters housing children and youth, eligible after-school care programs for youth, and nonresidential day care centers. This program is administered in most states by the state educational agency. A list of the state agencies administering this program is located at www.fns.usda .gov/cnd/Contacts/StateDirectory.htm.

The primary goal of the CACFP is to improve the diets of children twelve years of age or younger. Children fifteen and under from families of migrant workers are also eligible, and certain disabled persons, regardless of age, may receive CACFP meals if they are enrolled in a center that primarily serves people eighteen years of age or younger. In at-risk after-school care centers and emergency homeless shelters, school-age children are eligible to participate through age eighteen. Institutions that may participate in the CACFP include child care centers, day care homes, outside-of-school-hours care centers, at-risk after-school care programs, and emergency homeless shelters.

### Child Care Centers

Eligible public, private nonprofit, or for-profit child care centers, outside-of-school-hours care centers, Head Start programs, and other institutions that are licensed or approved to provide nonresidential day care services may participate in CACFP. Please refer to your state agency, as restrictions apply to for-profit institutions and institutions not required to be licensed.

## Day Care Homes

Child and adult group day care homes may participate in the program through an institution (a sponsoring organization) approved to sponsor day care home providers. The provider must sign an agreement with a sponsoring organization to participate in CACFP, since the sponsoring organization is responsible for the program administration. Reimbursement for meals served in day care homes is based on eligibility for tier I rates (which target higher levels of reimbursement to low-income areas, providers, or children) or lower tier II rates. The day care home must be licensed, certified, or approved by a local authority for day care services. Please refer to your state agency or sponsoring organization for further information.

## Outside-of-School-Hours Care Centers

Outside-of-school-hours care centers include public, private nonprofit, and for-profit licensed or approved institutions that provide organized nonresidential child care services to enrolled children outside of school hours and are distinct from extracurricular programs organized primarily for scholastic, cultural, and athletic purposes. Outside-of-school-hours child care centers operate outside of school hours and on weekends, holidays, and during school vacations. These institutions do not need to be licensed to participate in the CACFP, unless a state or local requirement for licensing this type of facility exists. If licensure is not required, certain health and safety standards must be met and documented. Please refer to your state agency for further information.

## At-Risk After-School Care Programs

At-risk after-school care programs are public, private nonprofit, or for-profit community-based programs that provide nonresidential care to children and youth after school through an approved after-school care program. The program must be located in a geographic area served by a school in which 50 percent or more of the enrolled children are eligible for free or reduced-priced school meals; have organized, regularly scheduled activities; and include education or enrichment activities. These activities occur after the regular school day ends and on weekends and holidays during the regular school year. These institutions do not need to be licensed to participate in the CACFP unless a state or local requirement for licensing this type of facility exists. If licensure is not required, certain health and safety standards must be met and documented. Please refer to your state agency for further information.

## Emergency Homeless Shelters

An emergency shelter, defined as a site that provides temporary shelter and food services to homeless children (public or private nonprofit), can receive reimbursement for nutritious meals and snacks served to children and youth. Examples of these types of institutions include family shelters, domestic-abuse shelters, and other facilities whose primary purpose is to provide temporary shelter to homeless families with children eighteen years of age or younger. Eligible shelters may receive reimbursement for serving up to three meals (breakfast, lunch, and supper) each day to homeless children through eighteen years of age. These institutions do not need to be licensed to participate in the CACFP unless a state or local requirement for licensing this type of facility exists. If licensure is not required, certain health and safety standards must be met and documented. Please refer to your state agency for further information.

## Meal Reimbursement

Each institution receives cash reimbursement for serving meals to enrolled infants and children that meet the CACFP meal-pattern requirements. Institutions receive payment for these meals in accordance with the state's assigned reimbursement method. Each reimbursed meal service must be supervised by an adequate number of operational personnel trained in the CACFP requirements to ensure that the program's administration is in accordance with regulations.

The CACFP reimburses up to three meal or snack services a day for each infant and child when the institution adheres to the requirements set by the USDA. This can be a meal and two snacks or two meals and a snack per child, except in emergency homeless shelters. In order to provide well-balanced meals for infants and children that meet their daily energy needs for building strong bodies and minds, CACFP governs meal patterns and minimum-portion sizes according to age. The USDA CACFP meal pattern includes infants (age birth through eleven months old) and children from one through twelve years of age. Frequently, the state child care licensing authority defers to the CACFP meal pattern as its required meal pattern. Following are the infant and the child meal patterns.

## CACFP Meal Patterns for Infants and Children

### BIRTH THROUGH ELEVEN MONTHS

To comply with the CACFP regulations, child care centers caring for infants must purchase all required meal components on the infant meal pattern according to the different age groups in care. The infant meal pattern lists the minimum amount of food to be offered to infants from birth through eleven months. The infant meal must contain each of the following components in at least the amounts indicated for the appropriate age group in order to qualify for reimbursement. Food within the meal pattern should be the texture and consistency appropriate for the development of the infant and may be served during a span of time consistent with the infant's eating habits. For example, the food items for lunch may be served at two feedings between noon and 2 PM. Solid food should be introduced gradually to infants when they are developmentally ready and with the parents' instruction.

### Infant Meal Pattern

| Birth through 3 months | 4 through 7 months | 8 through 11 months |
|---|---|---|
| Breakfast | | |
| 4–6 fl oz formula[1] or breast milk[2, 3] | 4–8 fl oz formula[1] or breast milk[2, 3] When developmentally ready, 0–3 T infant cereal[1] | 6–8 fl oz formula[1] or breast milk[2, 3] and 1–4 T fruit or vegetable or both and 2–4 T infant cereal[1] |

| Birth through 3 months | 4 through 7 months | 8 through 11 months |
|---|---|---|
| Lunch and Supper | | |
| 4–6 fl oz formula[1] or breast milk[2, 3] | 4–8 fl oz formula[1] or breast milk[2, 3] When developmentally ready, 0–3 T infant cereal[1] *and* 0–3 T fruit or vegetable or both | 6–8 fl oz formula[1] or breast milk[2, 3] *and* 1–4 T fruit or vegetable or both *and* 2–4 T infant cereal[1] Or in place of infant cereal you may serve a meat or meat alternate, such as 1–4 T meat, fish, poultry, egg yolk, cooked dry beans or peas; *or* ½–2 oz cheese; *or* 1–4 oz (volume) cottage cheese; *or* 1–4 oz (weight) cheese food, cheese spread Or you may also serve both the infant cereal and the meat or meat alternate |
| Snack | | |
| 4–6 fl oz formula[1] or breast milk[2, 3] | 4–6 fl oz formula[1] or breast milk[2, 3] | 2–4 fl oz formula[1] or breast milk,[2, 3] or fruit juice[4] When developmentally ready, 0–½ slice crusty bread[5] *or* 0–2 crackers[5] |

[1] Infant formula and dry infant cereal must be iron-fortified.

[2] Breast milk or formula, or portions of both, may be served; however, it is recommended that breast milk be served in place of formula from birth through eleven months.

[3] For some breast-fed infants who regularly consume less than the minimum amount of breast milk per feeding, a serving consisting of less than the minimum amount of breast milk may be offered, with additional breast milk offered if the infant is still hungry.

[4] Fruit juice must be full strength.

[5] A serving of this component must be made from whole-grain or enriched meal or flour.

## AGES ONE THROUGH TWELVE

The meal must contain, at a minimum, each of the components listed in at least the amounts indicated for the specific age group in order to qualify for reimbursement.

## Child Meal Pattern

|  | Ages 1 and 2 | Ages 3, 4, and 5 | Ages 6 through 12[1] |
|---|---|---|---|
| **Breakfast** | | | |
| 1. Milk, fluid | 1/2 cup | 3/4 cup | 1 cup |
| 2. Juice,[2] fruit or vegetable *or* | 1/4 cup | 1/2 cup | 1/2 cup |
| fruit(s) or vegetable(s) | 1/4 cup | 1/2 cup | 1/2 cup |
| 3. Grains or Breads:[3] | | | |
| Bread | 1/2 slice | 1/2 slice | 1 slice |
| Cornbread, biscuits, rolls, muffins[3] | 1/2 serving | 1/2 serving | 1 serving |
| Cold, dry cereal | 1/3 oz *or* 1/4 cup[4] | 1/2 oz *or* 1/3 cup[4] | 1 oz *or* 3/4 cup[4] |
| Hot, cooked cereal | 1/4 cup | 1/4 cup | 1/2 cup |
| Cooked pasta or noodle products | 1/4 cup | 1/4 cup | 1/2 cup |
| **Lunch or Supper** | | | |
| 1. Milk, fluid | 1/2 cup | 3/4 cup | 1 cup |
| 2. Meat or meat alternate: | | | |
| Meat, poultry, fish, cheese | 1 oz | 1+1/2 oz | 2 oz |
| Alternate protein products[5] | 1 oz | 1+1/2 oz | 2 oz |
| Yogurt, plain or flavored, unsweetened or sweetened | 4 oz *or* 1/2 cup | 6 oz *or* 3/4 cup | 8 oz *or* 1 cup |
| Egg (large)[9] | 1/2 egg | 3/4 egg | 1 egg |
| Cooked dry beans or peas | 1/4 cup | 3/8 cup | 1/2 cup |
| Peanut butter or other nut or seed butter | 2 T | 3 T | 4 T |
| Peanuts or soy nuts or tree nuts or seeds | 1/2 oz = 50%[6] | 3/4 oz = 50%[6] | 1 oz = 50%[6] |
| 3. Vegetables *or* fruits[7] (at least two) | 1/4 cup total | 1/2 cup total | 3/4 cup total |
| 4. Grains or Breads:[3] | | | |
| Bread | 1/2 slice | 1/2 slice | 1 slice |
| Cornbread, biscuits, rolls, muffins[3] | 1/2 serving | 1/2 serving | 1 serving |
| Cooked cereal grains or an equivalent quantity of grain or bread combinations | 1/4 cup | 1/4 cup | 1/2 cup |
| Cooked pasta or noodle products | 1/4 cup | 1/4 cup | 1/2 cup |

|  | Ages 1 and 2 | Ages 3, 4, and 5 | Ages 6 through 12[1] |
|---|---|---|---|
| **Snack** | | | |
| Select two of the following four components: | | | |
| 1. Milk, fluid | 1/2 cup | 1/2 cup | 1 cup |
| 2. Juice,[2,8] or | 1/2 cup | 1/2 cup | 3/4 cup |
| fruits or vegetables | 1/2 cup | 1/2 cup | 3/4 cup |
| 3. Grains or Breads:[3] | | | |
| Bread | 1/2 slice | 1/2 slice | 1 slice |
| Cornbread, biscuits, rolls, muffins[3] | 1/2 serving | 1/2 serving | 1 serving |
| Cold, dry cereal | 1/4 cup or 1/3 oz[4] | 1/3 cup or 1/2 oz[4] | 3/4 cup or 1 oz[4] |
| Cooked pasta or noodle products | 1/4 cup | 1/4 cup | 1/2 cup |
| Cooked cereal or grains or equivalent | 1/4 cup | 1/4 cup | 1/2 cup |
| 4. Meat or meat alternate: | | | |
| Lean meat, poultry, fish, cheese | 1/2 oz | 1/2 oz | 1 oz |
| Alternate protein products[5] | 1/2 oz | 1/2 oz | 1 oz |
| Egg (large)[9] | 1/2 egg | 1/2 egg | 1/2 egg |
| Cooked dry beans or peas | 1/8 cup | 1/8 cup | 1/4 cup |
| Peanut butter or other nut or seed butter | 1 T | 1 T | 2 T |
| Peanuts or soy nuts or tree nuts or seeds | 1/2 oz | 1/2 oz | 1 oz |
| Yogurt, plain or flavored, unsweetened or sweetened | 2 oz or 1/4 cup | 2 oz or 1/4 cup | 4 oz or 1/2 cup |

[1] Youth ages thirteen through eighteen must be served minimum or larger portion sizes than those specified for ages six through twelve.

[2] Must be full-strength fruit or vegetable juice.

[3] Bread, pasta, or noodle products and cereal grains shall be whole-grain or enriched. Cornbread, biscuits, rolls, and muffins shall be made with whole-grain or enriched meal or flour.

[4] Provide either volume (cup) or weight (ounces), whichever is less.

[5] Alternate protein products may be used as acceptable meat alternates if they meet the requirements specified in federal regulations.

[6] No more than 50 percent of the requirement shall be met with tree nuts or seeds. Tree nuts and seeds shall be combined with another meat or meat alternates to fulfill the requirement. For the purpose of determining combinations, one ounce of nuts or seeds is equal to one ounce of cooked lean meat, poultry, or fish.

[7] Serve two or more kinds of vegetables or fruits. Full-strength vegetable or fruit juice may be counted as meeting not more than one-half of this requirement.

[8] Juice may not be served when milk is the only other component.

[9] One-half of an egg meets the required minimum amount (one ounce or less) of meat alternate.

## Record-Keeping Requirements

Each institution must maintain records to support the reimbursement for meals served to enrolled infants and children. Records must be maintained for the current federal fiscal year (October through September) plus the three previous federal fiscal years, except when an audit is in process, at which time the audit records must be maintained until the completion of the audit. The record-keeping requirements include, but are not limited to 1) documentation of enrollment for all infants and children, including information used to determine eligibility for free or reduced-price meals; 2) the number of meals prepared or delivered for each meal service; 3) daily menu and production records for each meal service; 4) the number of meals served to enrolled infants and children at each site; 5) the number of enrolled eligible infants and children in attendance during each meal service; and 6) the number of meals served to adults. Refer to www.fns.usda.gov/cnd/Contacts/StateDirectory.htm for your state agency policies and procedures.

## Educational Opportunities

The USDA Food and Nutrition Service has resources and publications to assist child care providers in teaching children about healthy eating. Team Nutrition, Healthy Meals Resource System, and the National Food Service Management Institute have published resources that include nutrition newsletters, menu planners, and child care recipes. These and additional publications can be found at the USDA Food and Nutrition Services Web page on CACFP at www.fns.usda.gov/cnd/care/Publications/tools.htm.

## WIC

Institutions participating in the CACFP must provide each enrolled infant's or child's parent, guardian, or adult household member with information concerning the Special Supplemental Nutrition Program for Women, Infants, and Children (WIC). The purpose of WIC is to promote and maintain the health and well-being of economically disadvantaged, nutritionally at-risk pregnant, breast-feeding, and postpartum women; infants; and children up to age five. WIC provides supplemental nutritious foods, nutrition and breast-feeding information, as well as referral to other health and nutrition services. For further information, contact your state WIC agency at www.fns.usda.gov/wic.

## Further Reading

Gronlund, Gaye, and Marlyn James. 2006. *Early learning standards and staff development: Best practices in the face of change.* St. Paul, MN: Redleaf Press.

NAEYC. 2004. *Spotlight on young children and assessment.* Washington, DC: National Association for the Education of Young Children.

National Child Care Information and Technical Assistance Center. http://nccic.acf.hhs.gov.

Riley, Dave, Mary A. Carns, Joan Klinkner, Ann Ramminger, and Colette Sisco. 2009. *Intellectual development: Connecting science and practice in early childhood settings.* St. Paul, MN: Redleaf Press.

Riley, Dave, Robert R. San Juan, Joan Klinkner, and Ann Ramminger. 2008. *Social and emotional development: Connecting science and practice in early childhood settings.* St. Paul, MN: Redleaf Press.

State of Florida Agency for Workforce Innovation. Early Learning Services. www.floridajobs.org/earlylearning.

Wisconsin Department of Public Instruction. 2008. *Wisconsin Model Early Learning Standards.* Bulletin No. 08065. 2nd ed. Madison, WI: Wisconsin Department of Public Instruction. www.collaboratingpartners.com/earlyls_docs.htm.

## Web Sites

The following USDA Food and Nutrition Service Web pages provide more information on nutrition programs for young children and families.

Child Nutrition Programs state agency contact information: www.fns.usda .gov/cnd/Contacts/StateDirectory.htm.

CACFP educational resources: www.fns.usda.gov/cnd/care/Publications/tools .htm.

# Example of a Head Start Program's Meal Plan

**Date:** _____  **Center:** _____  **NSP or CA:** _____

| Meal | Menu Items Birth to 3 Months | Menu Items 4 to 7 Months | Menu Items 8 to 11 Months | Menu Items 1 to 2 Years Old (whole milk) 2 to 3 Years Old (1% milk) | Menu Items 3 to 5 Years Old (1% milk) |
|---|---|---|---|---|---|
| **Monday** | | | | | |
| Breakfast | 4–6 oz of breast milk or formula | 4–8 oz of breast milk or formula<br>0–3 T infant cereal | 6–8 oz breast milk or formula<br>2–4 T infant cereal<br>1–4 T applesauce (plain) | Strawberries<br>Multi-grain toast<br>Hard cooked egg<br>Milk | Strawberries<br>Multi-grain toast<br>Hard cooked egg<br>Milk |
| Lunch | 4–6 oz of breast milk or formula | 4–8 oz of breast milk or formula<br>0–3 T infant cereal<br>0–3 T mashed beans | 6–8 oz breast milk or formula<br>2–4 T infant cereal *or*<br>1–4 T pears softened and peeled<br>*and*<br>1–4 T beans | Bean and pasta soup<br>Lettuce/spinach salad<br>w/ ranch dressing<br>Crusty italian bread<br>Fresh pears<br>Milk | Bean and pasta soup<br>Lettuce/spinach salad<br>w/ ranch dressing<br>Crusty italian bread<br>Fresh pears<br>Milk |
| Snack | 4–6 oz of breast milk or formula | 4–8 oz of breast milk or formula | 2–4 oz breast milk or formula<br>1–4 T cheddar cheese<br>0–2 Saltine crackers | Lowfat cream cheese<br>Saltine crackers<br>Milk | Celery w/ sunflower butter and raisins<br>Saltine crackers<br>Milk |

| Meal | Menu Items Birth to 3 Months | Menu Items 4 to 7 Months | Menu Items 8 to 11 Months | Menu Items 1 to 2 Years Old (whole milk) 2 to 3 Years Old (1% milk) | Menu Items 3 to 5 Years Old (1% milk) |
|---|---|---|---|---|---|
| **Tuesday** | | | | | |
| Breakfast | 4–6 oz of breast milk or formula | 4–8 oz of breast milk or formula<br>0–3 T infant cereal | 6–8 oz breast milk or formula<br>2–4 T infant cereal<br>1–4 T banana, mashed | Bananas<br>Lemon poppyseed muffins<br>Milk | Bananas<br>Lemon poppyseed muffins<br>Milk |
| Lunch | 4–6 oz of breast milk or formula | 4–8 oz of breast milk or formula<br>0–3 T infant cereal<br>0–3 T peaches, mashed | 6–8 oz breast milk or formula<br>2–4 T infant cereal or<br>1–4 T ground beef<br>and<br>1–4 T green beans | Spaghetti w/ meat sauce<br>Lettuce salad w/ carrots<br>Vienna bread<br>Peaches<br>Milk | Spaghetti w/ meat sauce<br>Lettuce salad w/ carrots<br>Vienna bread<br>Peaches<br>Milk |
| Snack | 4–6 oz of breast milk or formula | 4–8 oz of breast milk or formula | 2–4 oz breast milk or formula<br>1–4 T peaches (diced small)<br>0–½ Sliced toasted bread | Peeled orange pieces<br>Bread sticks (soft)<br>Milk | Oranges<br>Bread sticks (soft)<br>Milk |

| Meal | Menu Items Birth to 3 Months | Menu Items 4 to 7 Months | Menu Items 8 to 11 Months | Menu Items 1 to 2 Years Old (whole milk) 2 to 3 Years Old (1% milk) | Menu Items 3 to 5 Years Old (1% milk) |
|---|---|---|---|---|---|
| **Wednesday** | | | | | |
| Breakfast | 4–6 oz of breast milk or formula | 4–8 oz of breast milk or formula<br>0–3 T infant cereal | 6–8 oz breast milk or formula<br>2–4 T infant cereal<br>1–4 T banana, cut | 100% Orange juice<br>Wheat english muffin<br>Milk | 100% Orange juice<br>Wheat english muffin<br>Milk |
| Lunch | 4–6 oz of breast milk or formula | 4–8 oz of breast milk or formula<br>0–3 T infant cereal<br>0–3 T mashed potatoes | 6–8 oz breast milk or formula<br>2–4 T infant cereal or ½–2 oz turkey and 1–4 T mashed potatoes | Roasted turkey<br>Mashed potatoes<br>Cooked broccoli<br>Whole wheat dinner roll<br>Milk | Roasted turkey<br>Mashed potatoes<br>Cooked broccoli<br>Whole wheat dinner roll<br>Milk |
| Snack | 4–6 oz of breast milk or formula | 4–8 oz of breast milk or formula | 2–4 oz breast milk or formula<br>0–2 Ritz crackers<br>1–4 T cooked, cut carrots | Baby carrots, parboiled<br>Wheat Ritz crackers<br>Milk | Baby carrots and dip<br>Wheat Ritz crackers<br>Milk |

| Meal | Menu Items Birth to 3 Months | Menu Items 4 to 7 Months | Menu Items 8 to 11 Months | Menu Items 1 to 2 Years Old (whole milk) 2 to 3 Years Old (1% milk) | Menu Items 3 to 5 Years Old (1% milk) |
|---|---|---|---|---|---|
| **Thursday** | | | | | |
| Breakfast | 4–6 oz of breast milk or formula | 4–8 oz of breast milk or formula<br>0–3 T infant cereal | 5–8 oz breast milk or formula<br>2–4 T infant cereal<br>1–4 T pears, peeled and softened | Fresh pear pieces<br>Rice Chex cereal<br>Milk | Fresh pears<br>Rice Chex cereal<br>Milk |
| Lunch | 4–6 oz of breast milk or formula | 4–8 oz of breast milk or formula<br>0–3 T infant cereal<br>0–3 T applesauce | 6–8 oz breast milk or formula<br>2–4 T infant cereal or<br>1–4 T chicken, diced small<br>and<br>1–4 T apples, peeled and diced | Baked chicken breasts<br>Corn<br>Apples chunks with strawberry yogurt<br>Wheat bread and butter<br>Milk | Baked chicken breasts<br>Corn<br>Apple chunks with strawberry yogurt<br>Wheat bread and butter<br>Milk |
| Snack | 4–6 oz of breast milk or formula | 4–8 oz of breast milk or formula | 2–4 oz breast milk or formula<br>1–4 T applesauce<br>0–2 graham crackers | Pineapple chunks<br>Pumpkin oat muffin<br>Milk | Pineapple chunks<br>Pumpkin oat muffin<br>Milk |

| Meal | Menu Items Birth to 3 Months | Menu Items 4 to 7 Months | Menu Items 8 to 11 Months | Menu Items 1 to 2 Years Old (whole milk) 2 to 3 Years Old (1% milk) | Menu Items 3 to 5 Years Old (1% milk) |
|---|---|---|---|---|---|
| **Friday** | | | | | |
| Breakfast | 4–6 oz of breast milk or formula | 4–8 oz of breast milk or formula 0–3 T infant cereal | 6–8 oz breast milk or formula 2–4 T infant cereal 1–4 T cut honeydew melon, mashed | Strawberries Biscuits with cinnamon Milk | Strawberries Biscuits with cinnamon Milk |
| Lunch | 4–6 oz of breast milk or formula | 4–8 oz of breast milk or formula 0–3 T infant cereal 0–3 T melon, mashed | 6–8 oz breast milk or formula 2–4 T infant cereal or ½–2 oz ground turkey (well-browned) and 1–4 T cauliflower, steamed and chopped small | Chili (turkey) with cheddar cheese Steamed cauliflower Honeydew melon Cornbread Milk | Chili (turkey) with cheddar cheese Raw cauliflower Honeydew melon Cornbread Milk |
| Snack | 4–6 oz of breast milk or formula | 4–8 oz of breast milk or formula | 2–4 oz breast milk or formula ½–2 oz cheddar cheese ½–2 Townhouse crackers | String cheese Townhouse wheat crackers Milk | String cheese Townhouse wheat crackers Milk |

Menu courtesy of Dane County Parent Council.

# Preventing Food-Borne Illness

The most common sources of food-borne illnesses in early childhood settings are

- improper hand washing;
- improper cooling of hot foods;
- improper cooking and holding temperatures (see the temperature guide for hot foods that follows);
- infected workers;
- cross-contamination (for example, raw meat juices coming in contact with ready-to-eat foods).

To avoid food-borne illnesses in early childhood settings, follow these basic steps. For more information, see the National Food Service Management Institute Child Care Tips poster (available in English and Spanish at www.nfsmi.org/documentLibraryFiles/PDF/20080130054129.pdf).

- Thoroughly wash your hands with soap and warm running water throughout the day and especially when you are about to handle food. In addition, thoroughly wash your hands before and after eating, before and after feeding a baby, after changing diapers, after using the bathroom or helping a child use the bathroom, after touching children's runny noses, and after contact with any body fluids.
- Cook and cool meat, poultry, and fish to proper temperatures (see the temperature guide that follows).
- Clean and sanitize food cutting boards. This is especially important when you use the board to prepare other foods

that will be eaten without thorough cooking (such as vegetables for a salad).

- Clean and sanitize all food preparation surfaces and utensils with hot, soapy water.

- Follow directions on baby food jars, and discard baby food if the use-by date on a jar has passed, if an open jar has been kept in the refrigerator for more than two days, or if an open jar has been kept at room temperature for more than two hours.

- Refrigerate or freeze breast milk promptly, and discard any breast milk or formula left in the bottle after feeding.

- Clean and disinfect diaper changing areas after every use, and keep diaper changing and disposal areas separate from food-handling and storage areas.

## Proper Cooking Temperatures

The U.S. Food and Drug Administration's *Food Code* (2001) recommends cooking food items to these temperatures and holding them for at least fifteen seconds. Check with state and local health department regulations.

## Food Temperatures

Eggs: 160° F

Seafood: 145°F

Steaks and roasts: 145° F

Pork: 160° F

Ground beef: 160° F

Poultry: 165° F

Mixed dishes, stuffed pasta, stuffed meats: 165° F

More information on food safety is available from your local and state health departments, USDA's Team Nutrition, and the National Food Service Management Institute (NFSMI). We especially recommend NFSMI's easy-to-read twenty-eight-page manual, "Food Safety in Child Care," available at www.olemiss.edu/depts/nfsmi/Information/cclessons/fs_center.pdf.

## Important Note

Bloody diarrhea in a child's stool could be a sign of a very serious and sometimes deadly bacterial infection called *Escherichia coli* O157:H7 (or *E. coli*). Children who are not toilet trained are especially likely to spread this and other types of *E. coli* infections. Make sure a child with bloody diarrhea gets checked and treated by an appropriate health care provider. If *E. coli* is confirmed, ask your local health department for advice on preventing the spread of the infection.

# Excerpts from MyPyramid for Preschoolers

The USDA's MyPyramid for Preschoolers has up-to-date and reliable advice on nutrition for children ages two to five. Included here are excerpts of key information from the MyPyramid for Preschoolers Web site (www.mypyramid.gov/preschoolers/index.html).

## Whole Grains

According to the Dietary Guidelines for Americans and MyPyramid, half of the grains eaten by children and adults should be whole grains. When the words "whole" or "whole grain" are part of the name of the first item on the ingredients list, the product is considered a whole grain food. Oatmeal and brown rice are also whole grains. Wheat flour, enriched flour, and degermed cornmeal are *not* whole grains.

## Meat and Beans

Foods in the meat, poultry, fish, eggs, nuts, and seeds group provide protein, iron, vitamin B-12, and other important nutrients that are needed by children's growing bodies. Some items in this food group are unnecessarily high in saturated fat, trans fat, cholesterol, and sodium. Check the "Nutrition Facts" part of the food label of packaged foods to select the most nutritious products that fit your needs.

## Fruits

Serve fruit as part of meals and snacks. When fresh food is not available or convenient, canned, frozen, or dried fruit are acceptable. Canned fruits should be packed in juice instead of syrup. When serving fruit juice, make sure it's 100% juice. Whole or cut-up fruit has more fiber than juice. That's one reason experts recommend that young children's juice consumption should be no more than ½ to ¾ of a cup (four to six ounces) per day.

## Vegetables

All vegetables are nutritious. Serve dark green and orange vegetables often. Fresh vegetables are great when they are affordable and available, but canned and frozen vegetables are also great choices.

## Milk

Some children don't like milk and other children like it so much they fill up on it, leaving less room for important non-milk foods. Make low-fat and fat-free milk and milk products part of meals and snacks for children age 2 or older. Ask parents to give you specific advice from their child's doctor if they think their child is lactose intolerant or allergic to milk.

## Snacks

Snacks should be just as nutritious as meals. Examples of healthy snacks from each MyPyramid food group are

- grains: dry cereal, whole-grain crackers and tortillas, and bread products;
- vegetables: carrot or zucchini matchsticks (pieces cut into thin strips), bell pepper rings, cherry tomatoes cut into quarters, steamed broccoli, green beans, sugar/snap peas, avocadoes;
- fruits: thin apple slices, tangerine sections, strawberry halves, bananas, pineapple, kiwi, peach slices, mango, nectarine, melon, grapes cut into quarters, berries, apricots;

- milk: low-fat cheese slices or string cheese, mini yogurt cups, fat-free or low-fat milk (for children two and older), low-fat cottage cheese;

- meat and beans: egg slices, bean dip, lean turkey or chicken slices or strips.

## Extras

Foods and beverages with added sugars or a high content of solid fat are "extras" that add calories without sufficient vitamins or minerals. Preschoolers can have some extras, but too many extras (often served as "treats") crowd out the healthy foods that give children important nutrients and may cause some children to eat more calories than their bodies need.

Examples of extras are

- sugary soft drinks, fruit-flavored drinks, candy, pastries, cakes, cookies, pies, and ice cream;

- the solid fats that are found in foods such as butter, stick margarine, fried foods, sausages, fatty meats, and full-fat cheese. Biscuits and some desserts are also likely to be high in solid fats.

## Salt

Most adults and children eat too much salt (sodium). Highly processed foods and foods eaten away from home are often high in salt. Serve foods that are as low in salt as possible. That way, preschoolers will learn to like foods with a less salty taste.

## Activities

MyPyramid for Preschoolers (www.mypyramid.gov/preschoolers) has suggestions for food activities with children, including

- minibagel halves cut in half, placed end to end, and topped with a thin layer of peanut butter or low-fat cheese spread;

- English muffin pizza;

- sandwiches cut into cute shapes or decorated to look like smiles;
- frozen bananas;
- fruit smoothies.

# Sources of Information on Gardens as Learning Opportunities

## Early Sprouts

*Early Sprouts: Cultivating Healthy Food Choices in Young Children* (2009) is a book with research-based lessons to help young children become familiar with and enjoy fruits and vegetables. The Early Sprouts program received a Champion Award from the Acting U.S. Surgeon General, Dr. Galson, in 2008.

## Got Dirt?

The Wisconsin Department of Health Services' Nutrition and Physical Activity program developed a gardening program called "Got Dirt?" for school, community, and child care gardens. You may purchase the tool-kit or download and print a PDF version of it at http://dhs.wisconsin.gov/health/physicalactivity/gotdirt.htm.

## Garden Mosaics

Cornell University's Garden Mosaics Program addresses multicultural and intergenerational gardening. The content is aimed at older children (ten and older), but the gardening resources can be adapted for early childhood. Garden Mosaics is a science-based program that promotes intergenerational culturally diverse activities that are appropriate for youth education in community settings.

# Recommended Sources of Recipes and Menu Planning Tools

Berman, Christine, and Jacki Fromer. 2006. *Meals without squeals: Child care feeding guide and cookbook.* 3rd ed. Boulder, CO: Bull Publishing.

National Food Service Management Institute. *Menus for child care.* http://nfsmi-web01.nsfmi.olemiss.edu/documentLibraryFiles/PDF/20080225095731.pdf.

These cycle menus meet meal pattern requirements for 3- to 5-year-olds.

U.S. Centers for Disease Control and Prevention. Eat a variety of fruits and vegetables every day: Recipes. http://apps.nccd.cdc.gov/dnparecipe/recipesearch.aspx.

This searchable collection of recipes features fruits and vegetables as part of the "Fruits and Veggies: More Matters" campaign.

U.S. Department of Agriculture Food and Nutrition Service. 2008. *Food buying guide for child nutrition programs.* http://teamnutrition.usda.gov/Resources/foodbuyingguide.html.

This guide helps you buy the age-appropriate amounts of food and explains how each food fits with applicable meal pattern requirements.

U.S. Department of Agriculture Food and Nutrition Service. 2009. *Recipes for child care.* http://teamnutrition.usda.gov/Resources/childcare_recipes.html.

U.S. Department of Health and Human Services Administration for Children and Families. *Fit source: A web directory for providers.* http://nccic.acf.hhs.gov/fitsource.

This Web site links child care and after-school providers to menu suggestions, recipes, and other resources on physical activity and nutrition.

# How to Help Children Be Active, Inside and Out

As explained in chapters 1 and 2, physical activity that promotes health-related fitness and movement skills should be part of every child's day (see *Active Start: A Statement of Physical Activity Guidelines for Children Birth to Five Years* by the National Association for Sports and Physical Education, www.aahperd.org/NASPE). Thus, it is important to help all children be physically active on a daily basis. Be sure to include all children, not just the children who initiate active play on their own. Favor non-competitive games that help children enjoy active play, even the children who are not particularly strong or comfortable with movement that requires large-motor skills. Teacher participation is important and helps children learn that everyone is included. If a child is reluctant to join one activity, ask the child to suggest an activity for the next day.

Outdoor activities for preschoolers can include running, walking, jumping, hopping, climbing, riding tricycles, playing catch, skipping, playing tag, sledding, playing on an obstacle course, doing gymnastics, and taking class hikes. Recommendations for active indoor activities include dancing, treasure hunting, playing virtual fitness games (such as those offered by Nintendo Wii), and playing hide-and-seek, ring-around-the-rosy, follow the leader, and catch with softballs.

## Outdoor Activities

- Build something from sand or snow.
- Collect items such as leaves, nuts, and stones for an art project.
- Clean up an area with brooms or snow shovels.

- Play active, noncompetitive games that are fun for all ability levels, such as

  - Owls and Mice—a game of tag in which there are several owls who try to tag the mice as they run across a play area. Children who have been tagged change from mice into owls and help tag the remaining children, until all the children have been tagged.

  - Foxes and Rabbits—a hide-and-seek game in which half of the class are foxes trying to find the rabbits, who are hiding. When all the rabbits have been found, the rabbits become foxes and the foxes become rabbits.

  - Kicking and Throwing—children are divided into two groups and stand opposite each other, about ten to twenty feet apart. Using playground balls, one group kicks the balls to the other group and then the other group throws the balls back. There should be at least one ball for every two children, if not one ball for each child.

  - Station Activities—four to six different stations are set up around a play area. Two to four children move together from station to station, completing each station's activity. Sometimes the amount of time spent at each station is monitored, and the teacher may ring a bell or blow a whistle when it is time to move to the next station. Examples of activities at stations are bouncing a playground ball, jumping over several items of different heights, scooting on a scooter board from one marker to the next, riding a tricycle around some markers, and throwing a ball into a hoop.

A curriculum with age-appropriate outdoor play suggestions for children up to age five is available for purchase at www.sparkpe.org/early-childhood.

## Active Inside Play

Develop a variety of large-motor play bins for use inside the classroom on bad weather days. The bins may include items for music and movement, balancing, throwing and catching, as well as for hopping, running, and crawling. Play music that encourages movement.

Gather lightweight items that can be used while dancing to music in a variety of ways and speeds. With appropriate supervision, pieces of colorful nylon can be used as scarves; two- to three-foot-long strips of wide ribbon can become streamers; and small plastic containers with dried beans or rice inside can serve as shakers. For coordination and body-space awareness, collect small plastic hoops that children can stand inside, spin, pull over their bodies, and throw soft items into and through.

Use clean white cotton adult tube socks rolled into balls for children to throw through the hoops that are held by their classmates. Children can play catch with the balls or even play a pretend snowball-throwing game.

Children can do coordination and balance activities with small cotton beanbags. Teachers can demonstrate ways to balance the beanbag on their bodies and ask, "Who can do this?" Encourage children to think of new ways to balance the beanbags on different parts of their bodies or while moving in different ways. Bean-stuffed animals (Beanie Babies) work well as beanbags. Play different beanbag tossing games using plastic hoops laid on the floor.

For running, jumping, and hopping, set plastic circle bases around the classroom with space between them that is compatible with a child's natural step. Play games of follow the leader, hopping, jumping, running, and marching. Imitate the movements of different animals on the bases, such as leaping like a frog, flying like a bird, and swimming like a whale.

Provide items for simple, non-competitive relay races with children in small groups of two or four. Children can move across the classroom balancing a beanbag or another item on a spoon without dropping it.

Provide a cloth, spring-supported tunnel for children to crawl through and play games in. They can pretend to be moles crawling into a hole, for example. Teachers can call the children's names as they crawl out, or they can try to guess which child will come out next.

# References

American Academy of Pediatrics. 2005. Policy statement: Breastfeeding and the use of human milk. *Pediatrics* 115 (2): 496–506.

American Academy of Pediatrics, American Public Health Association, and National Resources Center for Health and Safety in Child Care. 2002. *Caring for Our Children: National Health and Safety Performance Standards: Guidelines for Out-of-Home Child Care,* 2nd ed. Elk Grove Village, IL: American Academy of Pediatrics and Washington, DC: American Public Health Association. http://nrckids.org/CFOC/HTMLVersion/Title.html.

American Academy of Pediatrics Committee on Nutrition. 2001 (reaffirmed in 2007). The use and misuse of fruit juice in pediatrics. *Pediatrics* 107 (5): 1210–13.

American Dietetic Association. 2005. Position of the American Dietetic Association: Benchmarks for nutrition programs in child care settings. *Journal of the American Dietetic Association* 105 (6): 979–86.

———. 2008. Hot topics: High fructose corn syrup and weight status. www.eatright.org/cps/rde/xchg/ada/hs.xsl/nutrition_19399_ENU_HTML.htm.

———. 2009. Position of the American Dietetic Association: Vegetarian diets. *Journal of the American Dietetics Association* 109 (7): 1266–82.

American Dietetic Association and Dietitians of Canada. 2007. Position of the American Dietetic Association and Dietitians of Canada: Dietary fatty acids. *Journal of the American Dietetic Association* 107 (9): 1599–1611.

Anderson, Sarah E., and Robert C. Whitaker. 2009. Prevalence of obesity among U.S. preschool children in different racial and ethnic groups. *Archives of Pediatrics and Adolescent Medicine* 163 (4): 344–48.

Aronson, Susan S., ed. 2002. *Healthy young children: A manual for programs.* 4th ed. Washington, DC: National Association for the Education of Young Children.

Beals, Diane E., and Catherine E. Snow. 1994. "Thunder is when the angels are upstairs bowling": Narratives and explanations at the dinner table. *Journal of Narrative and Life History* 4 (4): 331–52.

Benjamin, Sara E., Sheryl L. Rifas-Shiman, Elsie M. Taveras, Jess Haines, Jonathan Finkelstein, Ken Kleinman, and Matthew W. Gillman. 2009. Early child care and adiposity at ages 1 and 3 years. *Pediatrics* 124 (2): 555–62

Birch, Leann Lipps, and Kirsten Krahnstoever Davison. 2001. Family environmental factors influencing the developing behavioral controls of food intake and childhood overweight. *Pediatric Clinics of North America* 48 (4): 893–97.

Birch, Leann L., and Jennifer O. Fisher. 1998. Development of eating behaviors among children and adolescents. *Pediatrics* 101 (3): 539–49.

Birch, Leann Lipps, Diane Wolfe Marlin, and Julie Rotter. 1984. Eating as the "means" activity in a contingency: Effects on young children's food preference. *Child Development* 55 (2): 431–39.

Blum-Kulka, Shoshana. 1993. "You got to know how to tell a story": Telling, tales, and tellers in American and Israeli narrative events at dinner. *Language in Society* 22 (3): 361–402.

Branum, Amy M., and Susan L. Lukacs. 2008. Food allergy among U.S. children: Trends in prevalence and hospitalizations. *NCHS Data Brief,* October.

Briefel, Ronette R., Kathleen Reidy, Vatsala Karwe, and Barbara Devaney. 2004. Feeding infants and toddlers study: Improvements needed in meeting infant feeding recommendations. *Journal of the American Dietetic Association* 104 (January): 31–37.

Brown, Judy. 2007. *A leader's guide to reflective practice.* Victoria, BC: Trafford.

Byrne, Elena M., and Susan A. Nitzke. 2000. Nutrition messages in a sample of children's picture books. *Journal of the American Dietetic Association* 100 (3): 359–62.

Centers for Disease Control and Prevention. 2009. Facts about ADHD. Fact sheet, October. http://www.cdc.gov/ncbddd/adhd/facts.html.

Coleman, Gayle, and Shelley King-Curry. 2008. Healthful eating doesn't have to cost a lot. UW Extension News. www.uwex.edu/ces/news/cenews.cfm?ID=3202.

Consumers Union. 2008. When buying organic pays (and doesn't). ConsumerReports.org. http://blogs.consumerreports.org/baby/2008/06/organic-food.html.

Devaney, Barbara, and Mary Kay Fox. 2008. Dietary intakes of infants and toddlers: Problems start early. In *Eating behaviors of the young child: Prenatal and postnatal influences on healthy eating*, ed. Leann Birch and William Deitz. Elk Grove Village, IL: American Academy of Pediatrics.

DeVries, Rheta, and Lawrence Kohlberg. 1987. *Constructivist early education: Overview and comparison with other programs*. Washington, DC: National Association for the Education of Young Children.

Dickinson, David K., and Patton O. Tabors, eds. 2001. *Beginning literacy with language: Young children learning at home and school*. Baltimore, MD: Brookes.

Feeney, Stephanie, and Nancy K. Freeman. 1999. *Ethics and the early childhood educator: Using the NAEYC code*. Washington, DC: National Association for the Education of Young Children.

Felsman, J. K., and G. E. Vaillant. 1987. Resilient children as adults: A 40-year study. In *The invulnerable child*, ed. E. James Anthony and Bertram J. Cohler, 289–314. New York: Guilford.

Fiese, Barbara H., and Marlene Schwartz. 2008. Reclaiming the family table: Mealtimes and child health and wellbeing. *Social Policy Report of the Society for Research in Child Development* 22 (4): 3–18.

Fiorito, Laura M., Michelle Marini, Lori A. Francis, Helen Smiciklas-Wright, and Leann L. Birch. 2009. Beverage intake of girls at age 5 y predicts adiposity and weight status in childhood and adolescence. *American Journal of Clinical Nutrition* 90 (4): 935–42.

Florida Partnership for School Readiness. 2004. *Florida birth to three learning and developmental standards*. Tallahassee, FL: Florida Partnership for School Readiness.

Fox, Mary Kay, Susan Pac, Barbara Devaney, and Linda Jankowski. 2004. Feeding infants and toddlers study: What foods are infants and toddlers eating? *Journal of the American Dietetic Association* 104 (1): 22–30.

Fox, Mary Kay, Kathleen Reidy, Timothy Novak, and Paula Ziegler. 2006. Sources of energy and nutrients in the diets of infants and toddlers. *Journal of the American Dietetic Association* 106 (1): 28–42.

Francis, Lori A., and Elizabeth J. Susman. 2009. Self-regulation and rapid weight gain in children from age 3 to 12 years. *Archives of Pediatrics and Adolescent Medicine* 163 (4): 297–302.

Freedman, David S., Laura Kettel Khan, William H. Dietz, Sathanur R. Srinivasan, and Gerald S. Berenson. 2001. Relationship of childhood obesity to coronary heart disease risk factors in adulthood: The Bogalusa heart study. *Pediatrics* 108 (3): 712–18.

Freedman, David S., Zuquo Mei, Sathanur R. Srinivasan, Gerald S. Berenson, and William H. Dietz. 2007. Cardiovascular risk factors and excess adiposity among overweight children and adolescents: The Bogalusa heart study. *Journal of Pediatrics* 150 (1): 12–17.

Ginsburg, Herbert P., and Sylvia Opper. 1988. *Piaget's theory of intellectual development.* 3rd ed. Englewood Cliffs, NJ: Prentice Hall.

Gonzalez-Mena, Janet. 2008. *Diversity in early care and education: Honoring differences.* 5th ed. Boston: McGraw Hill.

Greene, David, and Mark R. Lepper. 1974. Effects of extrinsic rewards on children's subsequent intrinsic interest. *Child Development* 45 (4): 1141–45.

Hall, William S., William E. Nagy, and Robert L. Linn. 1984. *Spoken words: Effects of situation and social group on oral word usage and frequency.* Mahwah, NJ: Erlbaum.

Hetherington, E. Mavis. 1992. Coping with marital transitions: A family systems perspective. *Monographs of the Society for Research on Child Development* 57 (2–3, serial no. 227): 1–14.

Hobden, Karen, and Patricia Pliner. 1995. Effects of a model on food neophobia in humans. *Appetite* 25 (2): 101–14.

Hoff-Ginsburg, Erika. 1991. Mother-child conversation in different social classes and communicative settings. *Child Development* 62 (4): 782–96.

Kalich, Karrie, Dottie Bauer, and Deirdre McPartlin. 2009. *Early sprouts: Cultivating healthy food choices in young children.* St. Paul, MN: Redleaf Press.

Keller, Kathleen L., Jared Kirzner, Angelo Pietrobelli, Marie-Pierre St-Onge, and Myles S. Faith. 2009. Increased sweetened beverage intake is associated with reduced milk and calcium intake in 3- to 7-year-old children at multi-item laboratory lunches. *Journal of the American Dietetic Association* 109 (3): 497–501.

Larson, Reed. 2008. Family mealtimes as a developmental context. *Social Policy Report of the Society for Research on Child Development* 22 (4): 12.

Leahy, Kathleen E., Leann L. Birch, and Barbara J. Rolls. 2008. Reducing the energy density of multiple meals decreases the energy intake of preschool-age children. *American Journal of Clinical Nutrition* 88 (6): 1459–68.

Maccoby, Eleanor E. 1980. *Social development: Psychological growth and the parent-child relationship.* New York: Harcourt Brace Jovanovich.

Maslow, Abraham H. 1970. *Motivation and personality.* 2nd ed. New York: HarperCollins.

McClelland, Megan M., Frederick J. Morrison, and Deborah L. Holmes. 2000. Children at risk for early academic problems: The role of learning-related social skills. *Early Childhood Research Quarterly* 15 (3): 307–29.

Michigan Team Nutrition. 2002. *The Michigan Team Nutrition booklist: An annotated list of over 300 children's books with positive food and physical activity messages*. East Lansing, MI: Michigan State University Extension. http://tn.fcs.msue.msu.edu/Booklist.pdf.

Morrison, Frederick J., Denise M. Alberts, and Elizabeth M. Griffith. 1997. Nature-nurture in the classroom: Entrance age, school readiness, and learning in children. *Developmental Psychology* 33 (2): 254–62.

National Association for the Education of Young Children. 2007. *NAEYC early childhood program standards and accreditation criteria: The mark of quality in early childhood education*. Washington, DC: NAEYC.

National Center for Health Statistics. 2006. Prevalence of overweight among children and adolescents: United States, 2003–2006. Health E-Stat, April. http://www.cdc.gov/nchs/data/hestat/overwght_child_03.htm.

National Child Care Information and Technical Assistance Center. 2009. Status of ELG initiatives. http://nccic.acf.hhs.gov/pubs/goodstart/strategicplanning.html/.

National Food Service Management Institute. n.d. Child care tips poster. www.nfsmi.org/documentLibraryFiles/PDF/20080130054129.pdf.

National Institutes of Health. 2009. Food allergy. *MedlinePlus Medical Encyclopedia*. www.nlm.nih.gov/medlineplus/ency/article/000817.htm.

National Institutes of Health and U.S. National Library of Medicine. 2009. Omega-3 fatty acids, fish oil, alpha-linolenic acid. MedlinePlus. www.nlm.nih.gov/medlineplus/druginfo/natural/patient-fishoil.html.

National Scientific Council on the Developing Child. 2007. *The science of early childhood development: Closing the gap between what we know and what we do*. Cambridge, MA: National Scientific Council on the Developing Child. http://www.developingchild.harvard.edu/index.php?CID=148.

National Women's Law Center. 2008. The reality of the workforce: Mothers are working outside the home. Fact sheet, February. http://www.nwlc.org/pdf/WorkingMothersMarch2008.pdf.

Nicklas, Theresa A., Tom Baranowski, Janice Baranowski, Karen Cullen, LaTroy Rittenberry, and Norma Olvera. 2001. Family and child-care provider influences on preschool children's fruit, juice, and vegetable consumption. *Nutrition Reviews* 59 (7): 224–35.

Pliner, Patricia, and Catherine Stallberg-White. 1982. "Pass the ketchup, please": Familiar flavors increase children's willingness to taste novel foods. *Appetite* 3 (4): 353–60.

Riley, David, Robert R. San Juan, Joan Klinkner, and Ann Ramminger. 2008. *Social and emotional development: Connecting science and practice in early childhood settings.* St. Paul, MN: Redleaf Press.

Roopnarine, Jaipaul L., and James E. Johnson. 1993. *Approaches to early childhood education.* 2nd ed. New York: Macmillan.

Sallis, J. F. 2000. Overcoming inactivity in young people. *The Physician and Sportsmedicine* 28:31–32.

Satter, Ellyn. 2008. *Secrets of feeding a healthy family: How to eat, how to raise good eaters, how to cook.* Madison, WI: Kelcy Press.

Seeyave, Desiree M., Sharon Coleman, Danielle Appugliese, Robert F. Corwyn, Robert H. Bradley, Natalie S. Davidson, Niko Kaciroti, and Julie C. Lumeng. 2009. Ability to delay gratification at age 4 years and risk of overweight at age 11 years. *Archives of Pediatrics and Adolescent Medicine* 163 (4): 303–8.

Serdula, M. K., D. Ivery, R. J. Coates, D. S. Freedman, D. F. Williamson, and T. Byers. 1993. Do obese children become obese adults? A review of the literature. *Preventative Medicine* 22 (2): 167–77.

Sigman-Grant, Madeleine, Elizabeth Christiansen, Laurel Branen, Janice Fletcher, and Susan L. Johnson. 2008. About feeding children: Mealtimes in child-care centers in four western states. *Journal of the American Dietetic Association* 108 (2): 340–46.

Snow, Catherine E., and Diane E. Beals. 2006. Mealtime talk that supports literacy development. In *Family mealtime as a context of development and socialization: New directions for child and adolescent development,* ed. Reed W. Larson, Angela R. Wiley, and Kathryn R. Branscomb, 51–66, serial no. 111. San Francisco: Jossey-Bass.

Underwood, Paula. 1994. *Three strands in the braid.* Austin, TX: Tribe of Two Press.

U.S. Department of Agriculture. 2009. Discretionary calories: What are "added sugars"? http://www.mypyramid.gov/pyramid/discretionary_calories_sugars.html.

U.S. Department of Health and Human Services. 2006. Child Nutrition. In *Head Start Performance Standards,* 29. Washington, DC: U.S. Department of Health and Human Services.

U.S Department of Health and Human Services and the U.S. Department of Agriculture. 2005. *Dietary guidelines for Americans 2005*. Washington, DC: U.S. Government Printing Office.

U.S. Department of Labor. 2008. Quick stats on women workers, 2008. http://www.dol.gov/wb/stats/main.htm.

Wallinga, Charolette R., and Anne L. Sweaney. 1985. A sense of real accomplishment: Young children as productive family members. *Young Children* 41 (1): 3–8.

Wardle J., M.-L. Herrera, L. Cooke, and E. L. Gibson. 2003. Modifying children's food preferences: The effects of exposure and reward on acceptance of an unfamiliar vegetable. *European Journal of Clinical Nutrition* 57 (2): 341–48.

Whitaker, R. C., J. A. Wright, M. S. Pepe, K. D. Seidel, and W. H. Dietz. 1997. Predicting obesity in young adulthood from childhood and parental obesity. *New England Journal of Medicine* 337 (13): 869–73.

White, Lynn K., and David B. Brinkerhoff. 1981. Children's work in the family: Its significance and meaning. *Journal of Marriage and the Family* 43 (4): 789–98.

Winter, Carl K., and Sarah F. Davis. 2006. Scientific status summary: Organic foods. *Journal of Food Science* 71 (9): 117–24.

Wisconsin Model Early Learning Standards Steering Committee. 2008. *Wisconsin model early learning standards*. Madison, WI: Wisconsin Child Care Information Center.

# About the Authors

*Susan Nitzke, PhD, RD,* has been studying and teaching nutrition with a focus on consumers, families, and communities for more than thirty years. She is a professor, extension specialist, and chair of the Department of Nutritional Sciences at the University of Wisconsin-Madison. Susan has a PhD in nutritional sciences and she is a Registered and Certified Dietitian. She is an active member of the Wisconsin Partnership for Physical Activity and Nutrition (WI PAN), the Wisconsin Initiative for Prevention of Obesity and Diabetes (WiPOD), the Society for Nutrition Education (SNE), the American Dietetic Association (ADA), and the American Society for Nutrition (ASN). She is a mother of two grown children who gave her a humble appreciation of how children don't always respond by eating the way "the book says." Susan fancies herself to be a pretty good gardener and cook. When time permits, she dabbles in watercolor painting.

*Dave Riley, PhD,* began working as a Head Start Assistant Teacher in East Los Angeles in 1972 and has several years' experience as a Head Start educational consultant. He has taught at the community college and university levels, including the last two decades at the University of Wisconsin-Madison, where he is the Rothermel-Bascom Professor of Human Ecology in Human Development and Family Studies and the Child Development Specialist for the UW-Extension. His published research has investigated parent-child relations, parenting education, and early care and education, including two other books by Redleaf Press. He was the codirector of the Wisconsin Early Childhood Excellence Initiative and the Wisconsin Child Care Research Partnership. He is a father.

*Ann Ramminger, MS,* has more than twenty-five years of experience as a teacher, administrator, trainer, and consultant in various early care and education systems, such as Head Start, full-day child care, part-day preschool, the WIC Program, the NAEYC accreditation system, home visitation programs, and technical assistance organizations. Ann was part of the research and development team for the revision of the 2008 Wisconsin Model Early Learning Standards. She has a BS in early childhood education from the University of Wisconsin-Madison and an MS in Administrative Leadership: Adult and Continuing Education from the University of Wisconsin-Milwaukee. Ann is a professional development specialist, with emphasis on early intervention, parent leadership, and collaborative processes, working for the University of Wisconsin-Madison Waisman Center.

*Georgine Jacobs, MS,* has been a professional in the field of early childhood education for more than thirty years. She has a BS degree in Education, with a major in Early Childhood Education, from the University of Wisconsin-Milwaukee and an MS degree in Elementary Educational Administration from the University of Nebraska at Omaha. Georgine has served as the lower school director of the Brownell-Talbott College Preparatory School in Omaha; site manager of the UW-Madison Preschool Lab; family literacy coordinator for Verona Area Schools in Wisconsin; and director of educational services for Head Start in Dane County, Wisconsin. She wrote *A Home for Tamara,* a children's book describing the life of a homeless child that has been utilized by many Head Start programs. Georgine is an active board member of her local NAEYC affiliate and currently teaches at Kids Express Learning Center in Madison, with specializations in gardening, nature, and art programming for toddlers and preschoolers.

*Contributing Author Ellen Sullivan, RD, MS, CD,* is a supervisor for the Wisconsin Department of Public Instruction Community Nutrition Programs Department. Her agency administers the U.S. Department of Agriculture Child Nutrition Programs, including the Child and Adult Care Food Program, Summer Food Service Program, and Special Milk Program for child care institutions, summer camps, homeless feeding sites, and outside-of-school-hours care centers.

# Index